MOTHER NATURE'S BEAUTY CUPBOARD

is a complete guide to hundreds of beauty preparations made from fruits, herbs, milk products, grains, honey and other wholesome, easy-to-find ingredients. Recipes range from such practical beauty basics as lemon-based pimple and blackhead remover, mayonnaise facial cleanser, herbal dandruff remover, even a buttermilk mix to prevent peeling from sunburn and Madame Helena Rubenstein's own Brittle Nail Formula . . . to deliciously self-indulgent peppermint-tea baths, spice perfumes, geranium rinse, chamomile-henna hair coloring and gelatin dessert setting lotions . . .

You'll also find sane advice for special skin and hair problems, exercises, health and diet aids and money-saving, make-it-yourself, completely natural makeup!

A Cornucopia of Natural Beauty Secrets
by Donna Lawson
beauty editor and co-author of
Beauty Is No Big Deal

Mother Nature's Beauty Cupboard

by **DONNA LAWSON**

Illustrated by Roberta Sickler

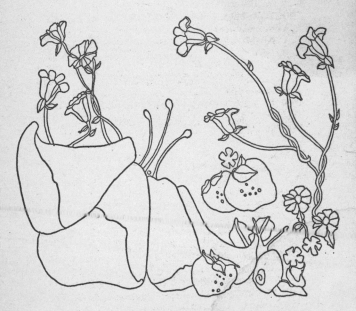

BANTAM BOOKS
Toronto / New York / London

MOTHER NATURE'S BEAUTY CUPBOARD

*A Bantam Book / published by arrangement with
Thomas Y. Crowell Company*

PRINTING HISTORY

Crowell edition published June 1973
2nd printing .... June 1974
A selection of the Cosmopolitan Book Club September 1973
*Selected excerpts appeared in HARPER'S BAZAAR, VIVA
and MADEMOISELLE*
Bantam edition published December 1974

For Jean Conlon, a blooming beauty

Contents

In The
Beginning
There Was Eve
and

This Apple

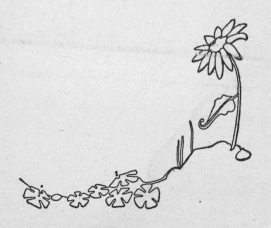

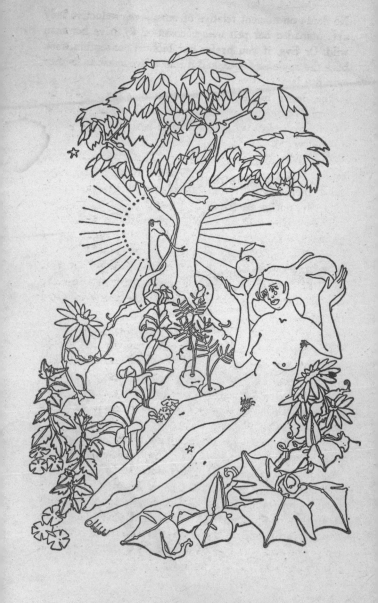

No doubt an ancient relative of ours, some seductive lady ape, pomaded her pelt with coconut oil to drive her man wild. Or Eve, if you prefer our biblical conception, took back the apple and squashed it into a face mask to further entrap Adam.

The desire to be more beautiful than even God intended has occupied women since time began. Whether this vanity is instinctual or cultural is a current topic of discussion.

So is the topic of natural beauty. That's what this book is about: beauty preparations made from fruits, vegetables, herbs, honey, and other good things that grow naturally, not in a test tube.

Today, when we are deeply concerned about the food we eat and the air we breathe, equal importance should be given to the products we put on our skin and hair. Not to say there are *no* good commercial beauty products. But who's to say? Unless you own your own chemistry lab, you can't know what goes into those pretty jars and bottles.

Sixty thousand Americans suffer allergic reactions to commercial cosmetics each year. Sometimes the effects are even more serious. Yet a powerful cosmetics lobby permits those products to go on the market without proper labeling. If you are allergic to any of the ingredients mentioned in these recipes, by all means don't try those particular recipes.

When you make your own cosmetics, there's no doubt what goes into them. Not to say a person couldn't be allergic to a strawberry or a lettuce leaf. But at least you'd know your poison. And could avoid it. Not every beauty preparation in this book has to be used, especially those that don't agree with you. You'd never have time nor the inclination to do so anyway. But if a couple of recipes or even one works for you, it's worth the price of this book.

There are many reasons, aside from ecological ones, to learn about homemade natural beauty preparations. For one, time has proved their effectiveness. Eggs, milk products, honey, bran, oatmeal, strawberries, the herbs rosemary and chamomile, these basic (as well as some silly things, as history has been no more immune to mistakes than we are today) have been consistently used through the ages. Our own grandmothers, their grandmothers, and *their* grandmothers made beauty preparations at home on the wood stove.

I learned to make my first natural beauty preparations in the blue-tiled California kitchen of a neighbor, a Parisian-born lady, who at sixty-five was still as delicately beautiful as a Fragonard painting. Violet leaves steeped in fragile china cups, egg whites frothed in crystal goblets, honey snuggled in ruby glass compotes. Mme. Albertine did nothing in small measure. Neither did her husband, Henri, who told of lavender-eyed yellow-haired folk from distant planets. I have grown up never having seen Henri's ethereal friends, although I'd never deny he did. Of the beauty mixes, I have more concrete knowledge.

While still a little girl I saw, to my astonishment, a violet leaf infusion, persistently applied, vanish a large ugly wen from my grandpa's bald pate. And I personally attribute my good skin to a regular use of Albertine's tomato and almond meal grains (although mine are not often mixed in an exquisite container with her special care). To this day, when in season, thin chilled slices of overripe watermelon, bunches of white grapes, and crisp cucumbers are kept in my refrigerator to use as moisturizers.

Albertine taught me to brew chamomile buds and pine needles to steam my face, to make a mouth wash from cloves and a hair rinse and face lotion from the herb rosemary (grown in my window box).

4

Over the years I've added many new recipes to Mme. Albertine's. One donated by a friend, Palavi Patal, uses a simple raw potato, known for years to East Indian women as a hand softener. Susie Olquin, a California friend, has sent me a poppy lotion recipe that she uses on her sun-dried skin. My Vermont friend Celie Fago has taught me to use pine needles to make a delicious bath solution. From Phaedre, in Woodstock, I learned to make a cologne with cinnamon bark and vodka. And recently Swami Harihardas, a graduate of twelve years' herbal study in his native Benares, gave me three recipes: a peanut flour hair conditioner, a citrus face mask, and a yogurt-based wrinkle-retarder.

Some of the ingredients in this book are astringent, or contract skin pores. Lemons and vinegar are fairly strong astringents; strawberries are milder. Other ingredients are emollient, or make dry skin and hair soft and supple. Bananas, avocados, olive oil, do this. Some products definitely reduce oiliness in skin and hair, like bran, which is used as a dry shampoo, or oatmeal, used in bath and facial preparations.

Sometimes ingredients have more than one use. Herbs, like chamomile, for example, do many things: enhance, prevent, *and heal*. Orris root has several applications, from reducing oiliness to preserving fragrances.

Not only do certain basic ingredients work, but I will also personally vouch that they cost mere pennies. This is important because of the initial saving and too because, not having chemical preservatives in them, homemade cosmetics spoil easily, must be chucked out, and must then be made fresh again.

But even with this limited shelf life, homemade cosmetics still save countless dollars. A fresh look at a cosmetics counter reminds you of this.

About twenty-five basic ingredients appear and re-appear in natural preparations, some as old as time itself. To me this consistency is a strong indication of their effectiveness. The ingredients for the beauty preparations in this book are easy enough to find. Most can be picked from a garden or tree or bought at any local supermarket or drugstore.

A few lovely and very effective components, some essential oils and herbs supplanted by "modern" products, are available only at old drugstores and herbal shops, which most large cities maintain for their historic charm. This is fortunate for a lot of smart people who still successfully use these places for medicinal and cosmetic reasons. Many beauty ingredients can also be bought at establishments supported by a whole new generation of people, quaintly, and for not-so-inside reasons, known as head shops. Check your local classified telephone directory under Oils, essential; Herbs; and Pharmacies (the pharmacies may have display ads indicating that they sell certain specialized products or that they have been in business for a long time). Probably there are such places near you; if not, obtain ingredients you can't find locally from the sources listed in the Appendix, page 171.

Read this book as you would a cookbook. Most of the recipes are very simple and inexpensive to make. Once you have the grasp of several ingredients and their performances, like any good cook you'll learn to change the proportions—take this out, put this in, and make the cosmetic that specifically suits you.

Remember that any time a recipe calls for a food product normally requiring refrigeration (eggs, milk products, vegetables, fruits, etc.), you should keep the mixture refrigerated. Do not keep such recipes for too long a time or they will spoil.

Money is a practical issue, certainly one of the main reasons for making your own cosmetics. But it's the love of nature that I hope will capture you most of all. There is a sensuality and beauty to tasting (they say any cosmetic you wear should be edible), touching, smelling, and sometimes watching your ingredients grow. And it's wonderful to see the effect of real untampered nature on your body.

Since nutrition, exercise, and massage are so closely tied in with the way you look and feel, they are discussed throughout the book. How skin, hair, and other parts of your body function is also described to make their interaction with the beauty preparations more understandable.

The recipes do work, as you'll see. That may be enough to know. But I wanted to know why and presumed you do too. So I've tried carefully to demonstrate why these preparations succeed and finally to tell the results to expect.

The book begins with your body, then gets into everything from face preparations to fragrance. But first let's look at the body, introduced by that famous sensuous woman, Lady Chatterley.

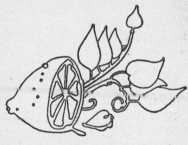

Body:
Salt Rubs,
Herb Baths,
and
Lady Chatterley

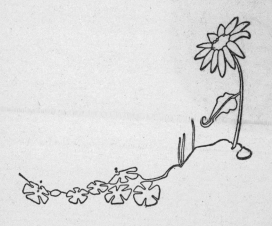

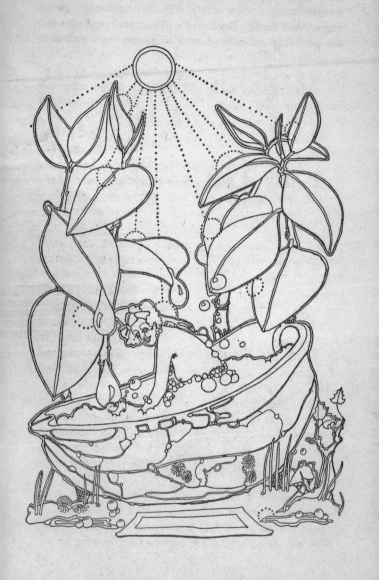

Lady Chatterley gave her body a long critical look while contemplating a love affair with her husband's game-keeper. And finding her flesh "a little greyish and sapless," she probably salt-rubbed it a soft rosy hue and then soaked in a bath of fragrant herbs.

This is my supposition, certainly not D. H. Lawrence's prose. However, in those days, although ladies concealed their bodies more, they did exhibit greater concern for them than we do today.

Today we liberated women race the clock, dash in and out of showers, and fall exhausted into bed; so it's a point of nostalgia to reflect on Mme. Jeanne Marie Tallien, from the French Revolution era, who daily stepped from a strawberry bath to be rubbed with a sponge dipped in perfumed milk, or on Marie Czetwertynoska, *belle amie* of Czar Alexander I of Russia, who bathed each morning in a tank of Spanish wine, later resold to the people. Wretched excess; ah, but what luxury!

Women thought so much of their bodies in Catholic countries that they even confessed while soaking in their baths. On second thought, the bath may have been a show of washing away guilt. Nevertheless, this ablution was called Modesty's Bath, although women received other callers, as well as priests, while sitting in their tubs.

Modesty's Bath

Combine 6 tablespoons crushed almonds, 1 pound ceunla campana, 2 tablespoons diced onions, 1 pint flaxseed, 2 tablespoons marshmallow root, and 1 pound spur-nuts. Pound all this together to make a paste and add it to the bath water.

The ingredients are archaic and very strange, since the bath was used centuries ago. But if it will help your confessions, better seek them out.

Not only ladies of leisure but working women as well

tenderly cared for their bodies. Dancers, circus acrobats, bareback riders, and women of unmentionable professions—job opportunities were limited then—massaged their bodies with deer fat to maintain muscle tone and skin texture. The following recipe was given by Lola Montez in her book published in 1853 called *The Arts of Beauty*.

Deer Fat Ointment

Mix 1 pint melted deer fat, 3/4 pint olive oil, 6 tablespoons white wax, 1 grain musk, 1/2 pint white brandy, and 1/2 pint rose water. During hunting season I suppose you could make this ointment yourself. Substitute beeswax, which can be ordered through most drugstores, for the white wax. Synthetic musk is available. The chapter on fragrances tells you how to make rose water (page 154).

Make this if you're either adventurous or a confirmed traditionalist; otherwise, use the simpler recipes for body rubs, baths, lotions, ointments, and liniments in this chapter.

BODY INSIDE AND OUT

All you put on the outside of your body won't help a mite if the inside isn't looked after first. By inside, I'm talking about general health: correct diet, enough sleep, relaxation, fresh air, and exercise.

A good book on nutrition goes hand in glove with one on beauty. Adelle Davis, the grande dame of healthful eating, has written several books on the subject. All will set you straight on food and how it affects your health and good looks. Should you not have a nutrition guide at hand, let me give you a brief rundown until you do.

First there's protein, which supplies strength and

energy to the body and which daily repairs and helps to produce body cells. A steak contains protein; so does a soybean. So a vegetarian can get enough of this good stuff if she plans well.

Carbohydrates in fruits and vegetables give a necessary source of energy; otherwise the protein supply would be called to work, leaving little left over to produce and repair body cells. But excess carbohydrates—the useless ones found in colas, candy, and cake—store up in the body's tissues, causing overweight. Bad news.

Fats are important for body energy too. Skin would soon lose its health and luster without them. Poly-unsaturated oils from fish, beans, nuts, and corn are good for you. But chocolate, excess animal fat, butter, and other saturated fats (generally, those that are solid at room temperature) are harmful. Body tissues retain them, making you fat. They clog pores and harden arteries. Who needs this trouble?

Ideally, enough vitamins should be found naturally in food. Unfortunately, as most of us are miles from home-grown food and have to settle for packaged, processed, and who-knows-what-else products, vitamins are often lacking. Supplements are necessary.

Vitamin A wins the skin medal. Eyes, hair, and nails also keep shiny and healthy-looking with regular doses of it. The Bs are taken to ease stress, a common ailment among "civilized" beings. If you are feeling generally out of sorts, doses of vitamin B complex will perk you up. Vitamin C fights infection anywhere in the body and builds strong teeth, gums, and connective tissues, the ones that hold bones in place. Vitamin D builds up the body's bones and helps prevent tooth decay. Vitamin E—wheat germ is the best source—gives energy, and it's said to increase sexual potency. It comes in capsule or oil form. The oil, used directly from the bottle, helps to keep wrinkles and scar tissue from forming. Pregnant women can help prevent stretch marks by daily rubbing the oil over their growing tummies.

There's more. Calcium builds strong bones, teeth, and gums; iodine helps regulate the thyroid, controlling metabolism, which effects your weight and the way you feel; iron raises your energy level; phosphorus makes hair and skin glow; sulphur strengthens fingernails and adds strength and shine to hair. Most vitamins and minerals are found in multivitamins, but some people prefer taking them separately.

Sleep? Your body tells you when it needs some. Eyes hurt, skin gets sallow, legs don't move as fast, a general

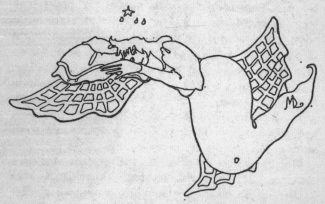

weariness overtakes you which eventually is taken to be natural. It's not. Go to bed when you're tired. Even a quick nap can revive you.

Relaxation can come in five-minute breaks. People save up for relaxation as they do for vacations, thinking it's something they need to find time to do. But getting your feet up is relaxing. A bath is like a short vacation.

Exercising, like relaxation, is often put off until there's time for it. Thinking about it as a rigorous routine can put you off. Thinking about the money it would cost to join a gym or a tennis club can put you off too. But exercising is running around the block or in your own back yard or jogging in place—anything that keeps your muscles used and taut and your bones limber. You can even think up your own routine of motions to limber yourself up.

Yoga is my favorite form of exercise, as it relaxes while strengthening the body. *Be Young with Yoga,* by Richard L. Hittleman, is a good book on the subject, taking you in small bits through easy steps. One of the glamour actresses of the forties, Marlene Dietrich or Gloria Swanson—I can't remember which—once said she got her feet over her head at least once a day. That's a good idea, you know, especially for most of us sedentary people, who either sit or lie down.

Once a day, if I don't do another exercise, a yoga shoulder stand gets my feet overhead. This way: Lie on your back with arms at sides, palms downward, so they press against the floor. Legs together, slowly raise them until they're at right angles to the floor. Keeping your knees stiff, your palms pressed hard against the floor, swing your legs back over your head. This enables you to raise the lower part of your back from the floor so it can be supported with your hands. Slowly straighten your legs and the rest of your body as far into a vertical position as you can get. At first hold position for one minute, then daily increase time.

According to Hittleman, and me too (because of the way it makes me feel), this posture aids weight control through its action on the thyroid gland, improves blood circulation, allows many vital organs and glands to revert to their proper position, and relaxes legs and other strained areas through releasing pressure on them.

Your body needs fresh air, and this is hard to find if you live in a large, crowded metropolitan area. I get more fresh air from turning on the air-conditioner than stepping out on the streets of New York when I'm there. Plants in an apartment help, as they give off oxygen and take in carbon dioxide. Getting to a park is also beneficial. But getting into the country, even if it means taking a bus to just outside the city limits, is my recommendation. There's nothing like a patch of green, blue skies, and a daisy or two to improve your physical and spiritual well-being. I'd wilt if Warren, Vermont, and Woodstock, New York, weren't there for me. I'd also be in bad shape if it weren't for a salt-rub bath or a soaking in fresh herbs.

SALT AND OTHER BODY RUBS

New cells are daily produced in the epidermis, or outermost layer of the skin. And daily they move to the skin's surface, die, and must be cleaned off, along with dirt, perspiration, and natural skin oils, in order to keep the skin's texture, tone, and color in prime condition. When dead cells stay on the skin's surface, it turns yellow or grayish and feels flaky and rough. Salt, papaya, and other body rubs roll off this residue, giving new vitality to the skin. Some of these rubs are very stimulating, others less so. They are a special treat in the spring and fall, after winter and summer weather have had their harsh influences on the skin—think of animals shedding their skins and fur. These rubs put you in tune with nature.

Saltwater Bath and Rub
This is usually used in conjunction with a salt bath and is very stimulating. Fill the tub and add 1 cup salt, swishing it around in the hot water so it doesn't settle at the bottom. Now you have a saltwater bath, with all

its refreshing qualities. In the middle of winter you can imagine being at the seashore. Wet yourself with the water, then stand in the tub. Pour a handful of salt directly from the container into your palm. Rub the salt over your body—shoulders, arms, buttocks, legs—in a circular motion, using more salt as needed. Do not use soap, although coating yourself with vegetable oil or mixing the salt with milk is okay if your skin is exceptionally dry. Salt awakens tired, dull skin and also revives your spirit. Two more benefits of salt: It's antiseptic and deodorizing.

Cornmeal Rub

If your skin is dry, apply mayonnaise or almond oil to lubricate it. If it's oily, just wet it. Rub cornmeal directly from the package along with the mayonnaise, almond oil, or plain water into your skin, making small circular motions with your fingertips. Stop when your skin feels

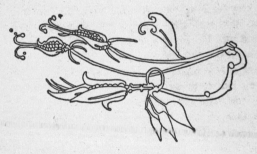

slightly flushed and warm. Remove the remaining cornmeal (with or without the mayonnaise or oil) with warm water. You may stand in the bathtub for this. Now bathe, if you like, or apply a lotion for a dry skin or an astringent for an oily one. The cornmeal rub stimulates and softens skin and evens up the coloring of a faded summer tan.

Oatmeal Rub

Taken directly from the box and rubbed on the skin,

oatmeal performs the same duties as the salt and corn-meal rubs, with this plus: It absorbs skin oiliness.

Cranberry Rub

Squeeze and crush fresh cranberries over your skin and rub in the juice. Let it dry (leave it on overnight, if possible, and rinse in the morning). The natural acids in cranberries have bleaching qualities that help to even out skin tone, particularly if you have a faded summer tan beginning to mottle.

Papaya Rub

Either fresh papaya or papaya tea (which often comes combined with mint) is fine to use. Mash several ripe fresh papayas until pulpy, then apply a thin layer to your body. Or use the tea bags (the mint gives skin a cool menthol feeling): Steep them in hot water, soak cotton pads in the still-warm liquid, and apply the tea all over your body (it's best to stand in the bathtub for this). When using fresh papaya, lie in repose with the fruit pulp seeping into your skin for about 1/2 hour. Papaya is rich in vitamins A, C, and K and in papain, a digestive enzyme that loosens dry, dead skin cells (to be discussed further in the face chapter [page 50], where this fruit is used as a skin "peel," much the way it is here). After the papaya has saturated your skin, rub it off with a dry terry washcloth. The friction rolls off the outer layer of dead skin. Mind you, skin layers are very thin, so don't fear large sections will come off, as when you peel from a bad sunburn.

Cucumber, Strawberry, or Peach Rub

Cosmetologist Christine Valmy suggests a nightly rub with fresh cucumbers, strawberries, or peaches when skin feels dry and irritated from general heat and perspiration or too much sunbathing.

RAPTUROUS BATHS: PEPPERMINT AND OTHERS

A bath is a small vacation, a chance to be alone, a solace against petty and good-size irritations, and a remedy for heat rash. Sometimes a bath even gets you away from the children. Kids generally hate associating with baths because it means scrubbing.

Certainly, baths clean you, washing away grime and flaky skin, but even better, they relax you. And they're sensual, like sleeping on a water bed, but you're floating embryoniclike *in*, not *on*, the water.

Some baths, on the other hand, are stimulating; a salt bath is. Sometimes a bath will put your body in gear when nothing else will.

There are baths to absorb too much oiliness and others to restore needed oil.

Strictly shower people don't have to give showers up in favor of a bath. Showering after a bath is a good idea— it gets off any soap film or flakes of skin the bath water might have soaked right back onto you. A shower can also create a sauna situation. First take a very hot bath, then if you have courage, dash under the prickling spray of an icy-cold shower.

Certain ingredients make water softer: the liquid from boiled rice, barley, bran, or oatmeal or a dash of regular market borax. These products in dry forms can be put into small muslin bags, important bits of bath equipment. The muslin for the bags is cut into 2 x 3-inch pieces. Then 2 pieces of muslin are seamed around 3 sides with tiny stitches. Oatmeal, herbs, or pine needles are slipped into the open side, which is closed with a rubber band or knotted tightly with a string. The lot is then tossed into the bath water.

As you assemble suntan lotion and sand pails for a trip to the seashore, gather the rest of your bath equipment: a shower cap to hold hair up so you can slide way down into the tub and not get it wet, a rough friction mitt (one that looks like it's made of hemp), a natural-bristle bath brush, a pumice stone to soften rough spots on the body, castile or glycerin soap, and any of the special bath ingredients coming up.

Ninon de l'Enclos's Milk and Honey Bath

Parisian Ninon lived between 1620 and 1705. It's said that even in the last year of her life, at eighty-five, she was ravishingly beautiful. She is famous not only for her beauty, which was extraordinary, but also because at one time or another she was mistress to practically every important *marquis* or *duc* in France; she was once kept by two gentlemen simultaneously. This distinction gave her great political power. After 1671 the lady retired from love on seven thousand *livres* a year. It's said her beauty was in part due to her famous baths. One called for 1 pint kitchen salt and 1-1/2 tablespoons bicarbonate of soda dissolved in 1 quart water. Separately, 3 pounds honey were dissolved in 3 quarts tepid milk. First the salt solution was poured into the bath, then the milk and honey. Into this beautiful Ninon would climb.

Mme. Tallien's Berry Bath

Mme. Tallien is famous for having married a prominent figure in the Revolution, Jean Lambert Tallien. If my sense of history is correct, he saved her from the guillotine before he carried her off to be his bride. Her bath was not very proletarian: Equal amounts (let's say 1 pound each) of strawberries and raspberries were crushed and thrown into a hot bath, turning the water a rosy pink. She emerged just as rosy, I imagine. As I passionately love berries, I'd rather eat them than bathe in them, but they seem perfectly reasonable as a bath ingredient. Strawberries, as you know, have astringent properties so this bath is probably best for oily skins.

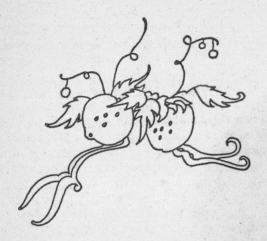

English Potpourri Bath

This was a favorite bath of that great czarina of beauty, Helena Rubinstein. People living in the country can pick the ingredients right from garden and field. City dwellers will need to settle for flowers from florists, herbs from window boxes or the supermarket: some lavender flowers, rose petals, and any other sweet-smelling herbs or flowers. Spread them out to dry and mix them with equal amounts of borax and orris root powder. "Place this in dainty silk or muslin bags with a ribbon attached," she suggests, "so that they can be suspended from the hot water tap of the bath. When the water is turned on, the bath and the whole atmosphere of the room become permeated with the compound, which can be repeatedly used before becoming exhausted."

Rosemary-Basil Bath

Mix 2 tablespoons dried rosemary and 1 tablespoon sweet basil in a muslin bag. Put 1 or 2 bags in a tub of very hot water. When the water has cooled a bit and the herbs have permeated it, get into the tub for a fragrant, refreshing bath.

Celie Fago's Pine Bath

Celie lives in Bethel, Vermont, with her mother, D'Ann, her father, Vincent, her boyfriend, John, two horses, a dog named Whiskey and another named Calhoun, a cat, and three kittens. And sometimes I live there too. Celie picks pine needles right from the trees that grow in her yard to make this bath. About 1/2 jar pine needles is steeped in enough boiling water to fill the container. The fragrant, stimulating liquid is poured into the bath when you want it. Pine needles can also go into bath bags, then into water.

Peppermint Tea Bath

Add about 1-1/2 cups peppermint tea to 1 quart boiling water. Allow the tea to stand for 1/2 hour or until it's cool enough not to burn your skin. Then strain it through cheesecloth into the bath water. This is a terrific cooler for both nerves and skin on a hot summer's day—so soothing, in fact, that it's been called the insomniac's bath.

OILY SKIN BATHS

Peppermint-Strawberry Tea Bath

Put about 1 tablespoon each peppermint tea and strawberry tea in 1 pint boiling water. Let it stand for 24 hours, then pour the mixture through cheesecloth before adding it to your bath. The peppermint is soothing; the strawberry has a slightly astringent quality, making it good for oily skin.

Oatmeal Bath

Oatmeal, as is, can be placed in small muslin bath bags, wrapped with rubber bands to keep them tightly shut. Or this more elaborate nineteenth-century recipe can be used: Mix together 1 pound oatmeal, 6 ounces powdered orris root, 6 ounces almond meal, 4 ounces shaved white castile soap, and 2 cups wheat bran. Place in muslin bath bags; this should yield enough bags to last a long time. Put 3 or 4 bags in the bath water at one time to soften the water and absorb excess oil and perspiration from the skin. Wheat bran alone put into bags serves this same purpose.

Bran Bath

Boil 2 pounds wheat bran in a large pan (a turkey roaster will do) of hot water. Strain the bran through a sieve. To the remaining liquid add a fragrance you like: 10 drops oil of bergamot, say, or 5 drops oil of rose geranium (see the fragrance chapter). Refrigerate the solution. Use it in the bath to soften the water and absorb skin oiliness, as they did in the nineteenth century, when this recipe was originated.

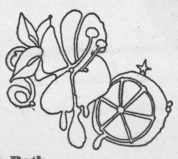

Lemon Bath

Squeeze enough fresh lemons to make 1 cup lemon juice.

Strain it, then dump it into the tub on a hot summer's day to cool your body, calm your nerves, and reduce skin oiliness.

DRY SKIN BATHS

Baking Soda Bath
Add 1/2 cup baking soda to a tub of hot water to cool and soothe irritated or dry skin on a sweltering hot day.

Peppermint Vinegar Bath
Put 3 heaping tablespoons fresh (if possible) or dried peppermint leaves into 1 pint water. Bring the mixture to a boil and simmer it for 2 to 3 minutes. Strain off the liquid and mix it with 1 pint cider vinegar. Let it stand for 2 to 3 days before using it. Add about 1/2 cup to a tub of hot water for a refreshing bath, particularly kind to dry, itching skin.

Cucumber Bath
Get the juice of cucumbers by slicing them unpeeled and boiling them in a little water. Strain the liquid from the pulp. Combine the cucumber juice with an equal amount of glycerin. Pour about 2 tablespoons of the mixture under the running bathtub tap and fill the tub. This restores moist softness to dry skin.

Glycerin Bath
Glycerin alone, about 1 tablespoon of it, added to bath water along with your fragrance makes a good bath emollient to soften and moisten dry skin.

BATHS TO CURE HEAT RASH

Laundry Starch Bath
Add 1 pound laundry starch to a tub of warm water to

cure heat and other skin rashes. Persistent rashes need a doctor's care, however.

Chickweed Bath

A tea of chickweed (supposed to grow wild in every locale in the world) added to bath water helps to heal heat rash and other body irritations. Order chickweed through one of the sources listed in the Appendix if you don't find it in your back yard.

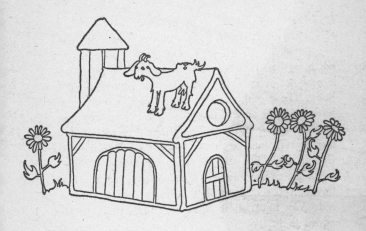

BODY POWDERS: CORNSTARCH AND OTHERS

Cinnamon-Cardamom-Cornstarch Hot Day Powder

Mix equal parts cinnamon, powdered cardamom, and cornstarch for a fragrant, cooling summer powder, especially kind to heat rash.

Plain Cornstarch Powder

The pediatrician told my friend Jean to use plain cornstarch on her baby, Peter, to prevent or remedy prickly heat. If cornstarch works on a baby's soft skin, it will surely help an adult's too.

Baking Soda Powder

Dust plain baking soda on the body to keep it fragrant and perspiration-free.

MASSAGE OINTMENTS: ALMOND OIL AND OTHERS

A massage is a luxurious gift from a friend. In fact, part of its relaxing effects is due to the interaction between two people. You *can* give yourself a massage, although not a totally satisfying one because of the physical problem of not being able to reach certain parts of your own body. These ointments are given in the hopes that you have a friend or will soon find one to massage you. You massage them, and most likely they'll return the favor. A terrific reference on the subject is *The Massage Book*, by George Downing. He recommends using oil for every massage, preferably a vegetable one: corn, olive, safflower, avocado. Nut oils can be used too: Almond, peanut. Any light oil is nice, especially if a fragrance is added to it.

Almond Oil—Lanolin Ointment

Mix equal parts almond oil and lanolin to make a thick, unctuous massage ointment to rub into the skin.

Jethro Kloss's Cayenne Pepper Liniment

In *Back to Eden* the famous herbalist Jethro Kloss recommends boiling gently for 10 minutes 1 tablespoon cayenne pepper in 1 pint cider vinegar. Bottled without straining, it makes a "powerfully stimulating external application for deep-seated congestions, sprains, etc."

BODY LOTIONS

For normal, dry, or oily skins, these lotions are to be used after a bath and at any other time to make the skin smooth and fragrant. The simplest lotion for all skin types is glycerin, scented with your favorite fragrance.

NORMAL SKIN LOTIONS

Lemon—Honey—Almond Oil Scented Lotion

Carefully blend equal parts (8 tablespoons each will do) strained fresh lemon juice, honey, and almond oil in an enamel or Pyrex pan over a low flame. Remove the pan from the heat. Bottle the lotion and refrigerate it. Rub it over your body to soften the skin and give it fragrance.

Ninon de d'Enclos's Lotion

Carefully blend 1 pint rose water with 1 pint almond oil. Stir in 1/2 tablespoon tincture of benzoin (a gum resin that can be bought at drugstores). The original recipe called for 5 drops attar of roses, an extremely expensive fragrance. Since it is used merely as a scent, drop it. This lotion softens the skin.

DRY SKIN LOTIONS

Vitamin A and E Lotion

Mix equal amounts of the contents of vitamin A and E capsules (a dozen each will do) by pricking them with a pin and squeezing out the oil or powder. Vitamin E, wheat germ oil, can also be used as is, mixed with glycerin. Add a few drops of your favorite fragrance. This works as a general softener on all parts of the body and is particularly effective on badly roughened elbows and knees.

Poppy Lotion

Poppies still grow wild in some places in California, where my friend Susie Olquin hunts them out to make a lotion for her fair skin, often dried from sunny days spent at Manhattan Beach. Take a handful of poppies. Put them in a small pan and cover with 1 cup boiling water. Cover the mixture and let it stand for 1/2 hour. Soak a cotton pad in the solution and apply it to sun-burned, irritated, excessively dry skin to soothe and soften it.

Cucumber Milk

This is a nineteenth century formula: Obtain 1-1/4 cups fresh cucumber juice in the manner described in the Cucumber Bath recipe (page 24). Make 6 tablespoons cucumber essence by mixing an additional 3 tablespoons cucumber juice with 3 tablespoons alcohol. Dissolve 1 teaspoon shaved white castile soap in the essence, add remaining cucumber juice, then 1/4 cup almond oil slowly, and finally 1 teaspoon tincture of benzoin. Put the mixture into an airtight container and refrigerate it. Shake it carefully several times over a period of 1/2 hour. Shake it again before each use. Rub the milk over and into your body to remove dry, dead skin cells and soften sun-parched skin.

OILY SKIN LOTIONS

Rose Water Skin Lotion

Add 1 tablespoon alcohol and 1 tablespoon boric acid to 10 tablespoons rose water. Bottle the mixture in an air-tight container and refrigerate it. Use this nineteenth century lotion on your skin to cool it, soften it, and remove excess oiliness.

Lime Juice Lotion
Mix equal amounts strained fresh lime juice and warm water. Apply this mixture to your skin with cotton pads. Do this while standing in the bath, if you like, so that the juice doesn't drip on the floor. The lotion removes excess oil, loosens dead skin cells, and leaves the body cooled, refreshed, and smooth.

SOFTENERS, LOTIONS, AND OILS FOR SPECIAL PROBLEMS

Orange Pulp for Neck, Shoulders, and Upper Back
Rub the pulp of an orange over your neck, shoulders, and upper back. The vitamin C content of the fruit, it's said, prevents aging of the skin and perks it up when it appears fatigued.

Almond Meal for Elbows and Knees
Make a paste of water and almond meal (available at drugstores, or you can grind your own from almond slivers). Work it into your elbows and knees to soften them and remove dry skin cells.

Grapefruit for Elbows
Rub the grapefruit pulp on your elbows to soften up dingy, dry elbows.

Honey—Lemon—Egg White—Bran Neck-Softener
Beat 2 egg whites until frothy. Mix together 1 tablespoon honey and 1 teaspoon lemon juice. Add to the egg whites. Add enough wheat bran to make a fine paste. Rub the paste into your neck, let it dry, and rinse it off with warm water. This softens a rough, dingy neck.

Wheat Germ Oil for Stretch Marks
Since our grandmothers' day, women have rubbed coco-

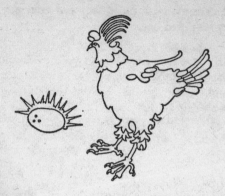

nut oil or cocoa butter over their expanding tummies to prevent the stretch marks of pregnancy. Wheat germ oil is terrific for this problem.

SUN TANNING: THE WHYS AND WHY NOTS

Dermatologists all agree that excess sun is extremely harmful, causing the skin to toughen and wrinkle prematurely. Melanin, the skin's pigment, which determines our coloring and how many freckles we have, is also the body's protector against harmful ultraviolet rays. Without melanin, your skin would burn like a wispy piece of paper.

Now, giving up the sun is too much to ask of anyone. We need some of it as a source of vitamin D. Besides, sun feels good—if taken in small doses. About ten minutes per day on each side is plenty for most people, fifteen the limit for very oily or dark skins. Even then, it's best to protect yourself against the sun with a lubricant. But if you happen to disobey, overdo the tanning process, and burn yourself, there are remedies to soothe the situation.

Other solutions even out faded tans and even give you a temporary tea-tinted one.

SUNTAN LOTIONS

Sesame Oil
Amazing sesame oil will stay on the body, even after you go in the water, until it's washed off with soap and warm water. Rub it all over your body to keep it moist and prevent burning.

Vinegar and Oil
Shake up 1 teaspoon vinegar with 1/2 cup olive oil. The vinegar promotes tanning, and the oil lubricates the skin.

TO COOL A PAINFUL SUNBURN:

Vinegar
Pat vinegar all over the fiery redness. The tannic acid takes out the sting. Soaking brown paper in vinegar and putting the wet pieces on your skin is a folk method of application recommended by my friend Sidney Shore.

Yogurt
Smooth yogurt over tender red skin to take out the sting.

Club Soda
Pour club soda over sunburned skin to soothe it.

Apricots
Combine mashed apricots with yogurt and apply the mixture to your skin to restore oil and take away the sting of a burn.

Pork Grease
Melt pork fat over a low heat (let it cool before you apply it) to make a soothing old-fashioned ointment for sunburned and generally irritated skin.

Baking Soda
When you're badly sunburned, spread a paste of bak-

ing soda and water over your skin to ease the pain. When it dries, rinse it off with tepid water.

Laundry Starch

Make and apply a paste, following the instruction above for baking soda.

Buttermilk and Tomatoes
Sunburn Peeling Preventer

Mix equal amounts buttermilk and mashed fresh tomatoes. Cover the burn with this mixture to restore skin oils and help prevent peeling.

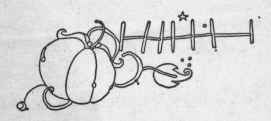

Cocoa Butter—Coconut Oil

Carefully blend equal parts cocoa butter and coconut oil —the amounts depend upon the area of skin to be covered. This ointment softens sun-dried, dehydrated skin and helps to retard peeling.

FADED TAN SOLUTIONS

Both buttermilk and lemon juice have natural bleaching properties. Marie Antoinette used to play milkmaid at the Petit Trianon Palace with her face, neck, and shoulders covered with buttermilk in order to maintain her fragile white skin tone. Buttermilk—or yogurt, for that —is left on the skin to dry, then rinsed off with tepid water. In fact, it can even be left on the body overnight to even out the appearance of a fading tan. Lemon juice, beaten with egg white to give it a stick-to-the-skin consistency, also bleaches and evens out skin coloring. This mixture has long been used to fade freckles, with some success, I'm told.

Quick Tea Tan
Stand in the bathtub and sponge your body with a strong brew of black tea. Let the solution remain on your skin for a few minutes, then gently pat off any excess moisture. This gives you a temporary tan tint, a terrific solution when you want to go without stockings in late spring or early summer, before you've accumulated a real suntan.

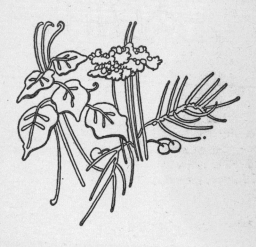

Face:
Almond Oil
and the
Wrinkle Treatment
of
Nero's Wife

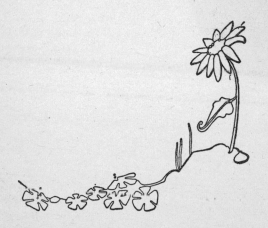

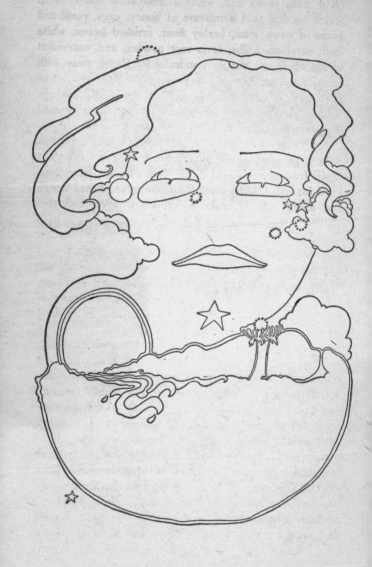

Ovid, born in 43 B.C., wrote a treatise on cosmetics in which he said that a mixture of honey, eggs, powdered horns of cows, gum, barley flour, crushed beans, white lead, narcissus bulbs, orris root powder, and excrement of sea birds was simply wonderful for doing away with freckles and producing a sparkling face. Just the kind of advice you'd expect from a poet out of his field; women died in droves from lead poisoning for centuries until they finally caught on to its deadliness.

Just because advice is old, it's not necessarily good. Nero's wife Poppaea powdered her face with dead-white chalk from the Channel cliffs. This couldn't have been good for her. On the other hand, she mixed bread dough and asses' milk to make a wrinkle-remover, and that couldn't have been all bad.

Just because a cosmetic is new doesn't mean it's any good either. Many "new" commercial skin creams have a mineral base, a byproduct of the refining of crude oil. The creams seem to penetrate the skin, but don't; they merely lie on its surface, never nourishing or moisturizing it. Using such petroleum-based creams for a long time will result in dried, aged skin.

Generally, if a cosmetic is edible, it's probably okay. But as most commercial products aren't labeled, you never know whether they are good enough to eat or not. I'd opt for the homemade over the store-bought cosmetic any day. I know what's in it, and as I've said, it costs me much less money than a fancy or even a not-so-fancy label would.

But there's more to beauty than what you put on your face, and I don't mean spiritual qualities. Beauty is literally not skin deep, as most makeup manufacturers would like us to think when they advertise their "perfect" products that *cover* all problems. Lovely skin doesn't start on the surface or even at the bottom of the skin's several layers. Skin is tied in with the workings of your entire body.

As your body functions according to the appropriate kind and amount of food, exercise, fresh air, sunshine, and sleep, so does your skin. When your body is in prime shape, its complexion will be too.

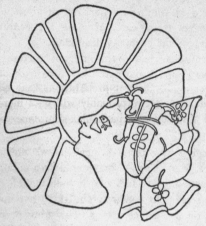

EAT WELL FOR GOOD SKIN

Many Victorian beauty books recommended eating green salads every day to improve the complexion. Whether the writers of those old books knew that leafy dark green vegetables abound in vitamin A, that terrific skin food, or whether they just luckily hit on a pattern of eating that made skin prettier I don't know. But the food you take into your body is as important as the food you put on your face. You are, as they say, what you eat—or don't eat.

Follow a good pattern of nutrition, watching your vitamin A intake by eating the yellow or carotene-rich foods—eggs, cheese, carrots, apricots, and cantaloupes—plus fish, liver, whole milk, and those leafy dark green vegetables Victorians gobbled to improve their skins. It's wise to take vitamin A in capsule form if your skin has been badly neglected; also take vitamins C and B, the former a general combatant against infection, the latter a buffer against stress, since both infection and stress are contributors to skin problems.

ABOUT SKIN

There are countless natural preparations that clean and condition the skin. There probably will be a mere two or three you'll need for your particular skin once you establish what type it is.

Generally, the categories of skin are broken up into normal, dry, and oily; the rate of secretion of sebum, the skin's own natural oil, determines which type yours is. Sebum gives skin its softness, moistness, and glow. Sebum forms an acid mantle on the skin's surface which protects it against external drying influences and bacteria.

Normal skin produces the correct amount of sebum and has enough cellular water retention to insure its own natural moistness. Keeping this or any skin type clean is necessary to remove not only dirt and pollution from the skin's surface but also the pile-up of cells that daily rise to the skin's surface and die. These cells must be gotten rid of to make room for new ones; otherwise the skin will become dull and lifeless and the pores will become clogged, so that the sebum won't be able to reach the surface.

Dry skin has barely visible pores, but it wrinkles faster than other types. The problem is a slow production of sebum, resulting in a lack of the protective acid mantle on the skin's surface. This is generally due to an improper functioning of the sebaceous glands. Another cause of dryness is a lack of water in the deeper cellular layers of the skin. These situations can be inherited, or they can be the result of poor health. Also, as we get older, these processes slow down.

External influences that dry the skin's surface are harsh weather, central heating, and the overuse of strong alkali soaps and dehydrating alcohol-based astringents. The balance of water-retention in the skin's cells can be affected by incautious dieting, which often goes hand in hand with decreased water intake.

The skin's balance can change, making a normal or even an oily type dry. Wrinkles are more likely to imbed themselves in dry skin, and moistness also keeps dry skin from flaking and becoming rough and irritated. So for many reasons it's necessary to keep this type of skin moist. Therefore watch your diet, drink enough water, and avoid the dehydrating influence of alcoholic beverages. Avoid overexposure to sun and other harsh weather conditions, or at least oil your skin to protect it against them.

Strong soaps and astringents should be avoided, although an occasional soaping with a mild castile soap or an application of a gentle lotion can't hurt the skin. In general, oil-based cleansers, lotions, masks, and saunas (the latter two discussed in the following chapter [pages 63 and 72] should be used on dry skin. Moisturizers need to be applied constantly to the skin's surface to make up for its lack of an acid mantle.

Oily skin produces too much sebum, giving it a shiny, large-pored, often sallow appearance. Overproduction of the sebaceous glands is the result of endocrine imbalance, a problem most acute during adolescence but also apparent during a woman's menstrual periods. Many women go through life with oily skins, and they're in luck in this area: Even late in life they are less likely to wrinkle. Wrinkles don't linger in well-lubricated skins.

On the other hand, oily skins are more likely to be victim to blackheads, pimples, and coarse pores. This is due to clogged pores, resulting from a mixture of external dirt and pollution mixed with the skin's own perspiration, dead cells, and excess oil secretion. Cleanliness is extremely important to oily skins to remove excess pore-clogging oils and the dead cells that cause the complexion to become sallow.

Oily skin should not be cleaned with heavy creams, since they block pores. Even natural vegetable oils should be used less frequently than on normal or dry skins. A mild castile soap or some of the milk products make good cleaners. Cornmeal and other cleansing grains are good to clean out the pores, as are the masks and saunas.

Lotions and astringents are also good for removing excess oil, although contrary to the belief of most oily-skinned women, strong astringents with too much alcohol in them don't remove the oil for long but actually make the sebaceous glands secrete more oil. Your glandular system is so smart that it will overproduce sebum to make up for the oil you've rudely removed. Milder astringents and lotions do the job just fine.

With skin that suffers from acne, there's a tendency to overdo the washings and use of astringents, thus removing the acid mantle so quickly that there is no protection against the germs that cause pimples. A smart thing to do after washing oily skin is to dab on a few drops of lemon juice to restore this acid mantle. It also doesn't hurt to use moisturizers on oily or acned skin, as they penetrate and nourish the skin, rather than lying on the surface and making it oilier.

In part, diet can control excess output of oil. So avoid oily, fatty foods: chocolate, nuts, fried foods, gravies.

41

Vitamin A can often help prevent blackheads and blemishes. When a bad condition persists, though, it's also best to see a dermatologist.

In this chapter are reliable recipes for various skin care preparations: cleansers, facial grains, peels, lotions, astringents, and moisturizers. As freckle lotions are traditionally included in beauty care books, I've listed a few, although I don't know why anyone would want to do away with those nice, healthy-looking polka dots.

The recipes to help specific problems—blackheads, acne, wrinkles, and so forth—are included with the general cleaning and conditioning recipes, as I believe that all are interrelated and that preventive care is far better and more reliable than a cure. There are a few cures included: a pimple lotion here, a wrinkle-remover there. But these remedies are far less important than getting at the cause of the problems.

SKIN CLEANSERS

Cleaning skin serves two purposes: to remove dirt and slough off dead skin cells and to soften skin. Many creams and oils can be worn at night. That business of night creams used to seem so mysterious to me, but it's just one of the many elaborate categories cosmetics firms make up to get us to buy, buy, buy. As far as I'm concerned, night cream is merely a lubricant put on the skin at night simply because you don't want to glisten with it during the day. Some people don't want anything on their faces at night. If proper beauty measures are taken during the day, you'll likely need nothing at night but a sheet. I hate to make the business of cleaning your face sound so simple, but it really is just that.

Vegetable, Seed, Nut, and Fruit Oils

For normal and dry skins, and occasionally for oily ones, natural oils that clean, soften, and condition the skin are purer, richer, and more nourishing than any skin preparation you could ever buy. And they cost practically nothing.

Safflower *Almond*
Corn *Avocado*
Peanut *Apricot Kernel*
Sunflower Seed *Soybean*
Coconut *Carrot*

Pour a little of any of these oils (wheat germ oil is rich in vitamin E, which makes it particularly good at retarding wrinkles and healing scars) into the palm of your hand. Use the fingers of the other to apply the oil to your face. Rub it into the skin in an upward motion, starting at the neck and moving toward the forehead. Gently smooth the oil under the eyes, starting at the inside, near the nose, and moving outward. Clean the nose by moving downward from the inside area nearest the eyes. Clean the forehead, moving from between the eyebrows upward and outward toward the temples. Clean the mouth area, smoothing the lines (if you have them) between the nose and mouth outward. Massage the oil deeply into the skin, then remove it with a dry terry washcloth. For skin that tends to oiliness, follow the cleaning with a mild astringent or freshener. When skin is dry, leave a slight coating of oil after removing most of it with the terry cloth. The cloth produces a slight friction, which helps to slough off dead skin cells. Apply a little extra oil to your skin whenever it feels excessively dry.

The Sacred Seven Oils
Skin Cleanser and Conditioner

Years ago, Gayelord Hauser began to use a seven oils mixture at his famous beauty farm. Now, a well-known natural cosmetics company makes a blend of seven oils that is sold in most health food stores. It's a terrific product, one you might want to buy. I've used and loved it. But I also learned how to make something similar if not exactly like it.

Combine 2 tablespoons each of safflower oil and sesame oil, 1 tablespoon each of sunflower seed oil, avocado oil, and peanut oil, 1-1/2 teaspoons each of olive oil and wheat germ oil, and 3 drops oil of your favorite fragrance (I use lemon verbena). I mix my preparation in a blender, although I suppose it could be put in a tightly lidded jar and given a good shake. Great as a skin cleanser and conditioner.

Oil and Herb Cleanser and
Conditioner

Herbs can be mixed with vegetable and other oils for variety, as a cleanser and conditioner. The herbs serve two purposes: They are cosmetic, and they are aromatic. Add a handful of crushed dried peppermint or some extract of mint (available at drugstores) to the oil. The natural odor of the oil should not interfere with the herb's fragrance—that is, if you want its scent. Safflower oil has little natural odor, so you might prefer to mix your herbs with it. Mint has a cooling, menthol effect on the skin, giving it a natural warmth and glow. Sage, known for its healing qualities, is another nice addition. My favorite is rosemary. A small spice jar of safflower oil with about 1 tablespoon of rosemary in it sits in my refrigerator to be used for cleaning and lubricating my skin when it feels dry. The rosemary picks up the color of my skin and gives off a slightly spicy fragrance.

The herbs listed below have several cosmetic benefits: They have antiseptic qualities, they stimulate and improve the skin's circulation, and they heal.

Lime Flowers
Fennel
Yarrow
Marigold
Nettles
Chamomile
Horsetail
Elder Flowers

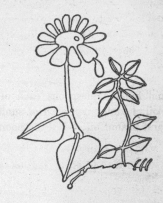

Avocado Cleanser

For skin that is exceptionally dry, avocado is an excellent cleanser and conditioner. Mash it thoroughly before applying it to the skin. Massage it in carefully for several minutes. Remove the residue with a tissue, but leave a coating of the avocado's rich oil on the skin. This is good to apply before going to bed so that the oil can penetrate the skin all night. Avocado is rich in vitamin A. It's also an ancient and primitive cleanser known to the Peruvians and Incas.

Strawberry and Shortening Cleanser

This cleanser is recommended for normal and dry skins, not oily ones, as it might clog the pores if it is not thoroughly removed with an astringent. Crush 4 plump, juicy strawberries. Blend well with 6 tablespoons vegetable shortening and 3 tablespoons witch hazel. Massage it into the skin and remove the excess with a tissue. Follow up with a mild freshener.

Cosmetic Mayonnaise

This is an excellent cleanser and conditioner for normal and dry skins. Mayonnaise has the cleansing, nourishing, softening qualities of oil, with the addition of egg yolk, containing carotene, vitamin A, and lecithin, which helps to plump up skin cells. Make your own mayonnaise or pull a jar directly out of the refrigerator and generously apply the contents to your skin. You can also add a few drops of lemon juice, an astringent and natural bleaching agent.

SOAP SOLUTIONS FOR SENSITIVE SKINS

Soap solutions generally have a slightly drying effect, so women who tend to oil up like to use them. This one is so mild, however, that even dry skins will find it harmless.

Almond Meal Soap

Mix together 3/4 cup almond meal, 1/2 cup rice powder (available at health food stores), and 1-1/4 cups shaved castile soap. Keep the mixture in a tightly lidded jar. When using this soap, make a lather with your hands by adding warm water. Rub it gently into your skin and remove it with warm water.

Turkish Princess Soap

As the name of this recipe implies, this soap was used by a Turkish princess, so a Victorian beauty book claims, although it fails to say which princess. Because of the oatmeal content of this soap, it's terrific for oily skins (oatmeal is absorbent). Shave very fine 1 pound white castile soap. Place it in a porcelain or glass pan and cover it with cold water. Place the pan over a low flame. When the soap is softened by the heat and mixed with the water, stir into it 1/2 pound oatmeal. Mix well. When the ingredients are thoroughly blended, take the pan off the stove. When the mixture has cooled so that you can handle it, form it into balls the size of walnuts. Or the soap can be used warm, in its liquid state.

MILK PRODUCT CLEANSERS

Milk and milk products, high in vitamin A, make cleaning agents for all skins, including oily ones.

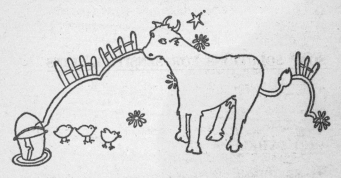

Buttermilk Cleanser
Buttermilk can be applied directly to the skin, then wiped off with a terry washcloth or rinsed off with warm water, followed by a splash of cold.

Yogurt Cleanser
Plain yogurt also makes an excellent skin cleanser, applied either directly from the container or with herbs added. Here's another idea: To get the extra qualities of vitamin A, a capsule can be punctured and the contents mixed with yogurt or any other skin cleanser. Wipe or rinse it off and follow with cold water.

Milk and Strawberry Cleanser
A cup of milk or fresh cream with the slightly astringent addition of a handful of mashed strawberries is an age-old Swiss skin formula. Apply the mixture generously to your skin. Leave it on long enough to allow it to deeply

47

nourish the skin. Remove it with a tissue or warm water, followed with cold water.

Sour Cream Cleanser

Cold sour cream is cooling and cleansing on a hot day. Apply a liberal amount to the skin and leave it on up to 20 minutes. Remove it with a terry washcloth, dampened slightly with warm water, then rinse with cold water. Sour cream is very stimulating to the skin's circulation, so it may be too strong for people with acne.

Yogurt-Cream-Almond-Salt Cleanser

Yogurt, cream, and crushed almonds in equal amounts and a pinch of sea salt placed in a muslin bag, then moistened and rubbed over the face, make a good cleaning agent for oily skin. Rinse first with warm water, then with cold. Follow with a freshener if you like.

CLEANSING GRAINS: ALMOND MEAL AND OTHERS

Cleansing grains, like face peels, are used to clear away blackheads, rough dead skin cells, and other troubles that keep the skin from being clean and smooth. They also stimulate circulation, picking up the color of sallow, tired skin. Since these grains are abrasive, they should be used with caution. When skin is sensitive due to too much sun, eruptions, or abrasions, they should be

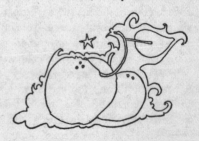

avoided until the problems have gone. Use cleansing grains on clean skin no more than twice a week, only once if they tend to irritate. Follow the cleansing with a cold water splash and a mild astringent to close up the clean, open pores.

Mme. Albertine's Tomato–Almond Meal Grains

Pulverize almond slices in a blender if you have one; grind or grate them if you don't. Mix the almond meal with an equal amount mashed ripe tomato. The acidity of the tomato rolls off flakes of dry outer skin, as it does in the face peel. Both the tomato and almond meal penetrate pores, clearing them of blackheads, especially in those stubborn areas around the nose and chin. Remove the mixture with cool water or wipe it off, leaving a coating of the natural oils and juices. This is one of my favorite recipes—works for me every time.

Oatmeal Grains

Mix dry oatmeal with water and rub it into the skin, especially in the areas where blackheads tend to collect: the chin and around the nose. Gently rub the mixture off with a terry washcloth and cool water. This mixture blots skin oils, as well as removing blackheads.

Cornmeal and Honey Grains

Mix 1 tablespoon cornmeal with 1 tablespoon honey. Gently massage this into those areas that need attention in order to remove blackheads and rough skin. Gently rub the mixture off with a terry washcloth; rinse with warm, then with cool, water.

Almond Meal, Oatmeal, Honey, and Egg White Grains

Make a paste of almond meal, oatmeal, and honey in equal amounts and one egg white. Massage it into the skin. The friction of the mixture removes rough skin and blackheads.

FACE PEELS

Facial salons advertise face peels. Thinking they must be formidable, the process resembling a third degree burn, I didn't want to think about them further. Investigation, however (as I am curious), proved face peels were very simple and certainly not threatening. In essence, peeling the face merely means loosening that top layer of dead skin cells and rubbing them off. Four peels do an excellent job of this: tomato, which is good for all skins; papaya, excellent for normal and dry skins (see page 18); lemon, used expressly for oily skins; and potato, which has healing properties for skins with acne. All peels should be applied to clean skin.

Tomato Face Peel

Rub tomato slices directly into your skin, concentrating on areas infested with blackheads. Tomatoes contain vitamin C, which has healing powers, and an acid that removes dead skin and unplugs pores, making skin soft and radiant.

Lemon Face Peel

Place fresh juice from a lemon and the fruit's grated rind in a glass bowl and let them stand overnight. In the morning, apply the solution to your face: Saturate cotton balls and lavishly apply the liquid to your skin. Let it dry, then rub the skin gently. A layer of dead skin cells will loosen. Remove them with a terry washcloth, then rinse off any remaining lemon solution.

Potato Face Peel

Raw potato can be rubbed directly over blemished skin. It removes dead skin and grime even after the skin has been thoroughly cleaned, and it has healing properties that go to work on skin eruptions.

LOTIONS, FRESHENERS, TONICS, RINSES, ASTRINGENTS, AND COSMETIC VINEGARS

Generally, lotions, fresheners, tonics, and rinses follow cleaning and remove the last remnants of the cleanser or soap. They have a refreshing, soothing, healing effect on the skin and can be used on all skin types, including dry ones, since the alcohol content, with its harsh drying influence, is minimal. Astringents and cosmetic vinegars are stronger, more antiseptic, and more drying due to their content of alcohol and tannic acid. They should be used only on oily skins and then not with great frequency. The first few recipes below can be used on dry skins, as well as normal and oily ones. The rest of the recipes, as will be noted, are reserved for normal and sometimes only for oily skins.

FOR DRY SKINS

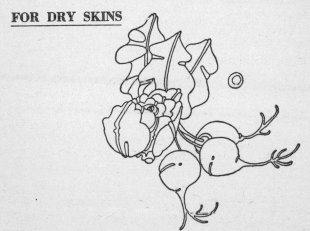

Beet Bath

For centuries, in China, Turkey, and Egypt women have bathed their faces in beet juice for the tonic effect, then rinsed it off with cool water.

Peppermint Rinse

Add 1 teaspoon crushed dried peppermint (or peppermint tea) to 1 cup boiling water. Let the ingredients steep for 1/2 hour. Strain off the liquid and bottle it. This same process can be followed with chamomile or rosemary. Use the rinse as a freshener after a cleaning.

Buttermilk Lotion

Combine 2 tablespoons buttermilk with the juice of 1 fresh tomato. Rinse your face with the solution and wipe off the residue with tissues. A nineteenth century beauty book claims buttermilk to be a general emollient, its daily application making the skin "soft, smooth, and white and preserving it from the drying of winds, cold, vivid sunshine and the like." It *is* the best lotion for dry skin.

FOR DRY AND NORMAL SKINS

Club Soda Freshener

Bathe your face in cold club soda to remove perspiration and refresh the skin on a scorching-hot day.

Honey Face Lotion

Mix 1 part honey with 9 parts witch hazel. Pour the lotion into a tightly lidded container and shake it well. Keep it refrigerated. Use this as a refreshing skin tonic.

FOR NORMAL AND OILY SKINS

Fruity Freshener

Mix 1 teaspoon lemon juice, 1 teaspoon lime juice, and 1 teaspoon orange juice with 1 cup yogurt. Smooth this over your face, then rinse it off with warm water, followed by a splash of cold. This tightens pores.

Eva's Mother's Strawberry Astringent

Eva's mother came from Czechoslovakia, where she grew up using crushed strawberries on her face for their astringent qualities. She taught this practice to Eva, who grew up in London, who taught it to me, who grew up in California. It's lovely to use this luscious fruit to refresh your face and tighten its pores on a hot summer day.

Vita's Mother's Cucumber Lotion

Vita is a wonderful woman who lives in Woodstock, New York, and gives marvelous massages. Her mother grew up in South America. This is her recipe: Extract the juice from a cucumber by first grating it, then pushing it through a sieve. Add 4 tablespoons juice to an 8-ounce glass. Stir in 1/2 teaspoon honey. Add a few drops lemon juice. Fill the glass to the top with 70% alcohol. Pour the mixture into a tightly lidded jar and keep it in the refrigerator. Use it as a refreshing skin lotion.

Cucumber Lotion No. 2

Cucumber, with its natural skin-soothing and astringent properties, has been used for centuries to tone the skin after cleaning. This recipe, dating back to the nineteenth century, calls for 3 tablespoons cucumber juice mixed with 1 teaspoon tincture of benzoin and 3/4 cup elder flower water. Keep this in the refrigerator in a tightly lidded jar to use as a cool, refreshing lotion.

FOR OILY SKINS

Oatmeal Lotion

Tie a handful of oatmeal in a piece of cheesecloth and secure it with a rubber band. Place the bundle under running warm water until it's saturated. When it's completely wet, apply the oatmeal package to the skin. Let the oatmeal liquid dry on your face for about 5 minutes, then rinse it off with warm water. The oatmeal liquid absorbs excess skin oil.

Lemon Astringent

Mix 2 tablespoons lemon juice with 1 tablespoon glycerin and 1 tablespoon alcohol in a measuring cup. Add enough witch hazel to measure 1 cup. Refrigerate the liquid in a tightly lidded jar. Use it to remove excess oil and tighten pores.

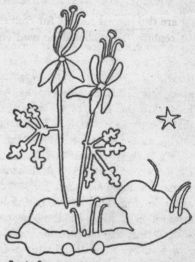

Rose Water Astringent

Add 3/4 cup rose water (see page 154 for the recipe) to 1/4 cup witch hazel. Stir in 1 teaspoon honey, 1/2 teaspoon white vinegar, a pinch of alum (available at drugstores), 1/2 teaspoon glycerin, 1/2 teaspoon spirits of camphor, and 1/2 teaspoon extract of mint. Refrigerate this in a tightly lidded jar. Shake it well before using it. This nineteenth century preparation removes excess skin oil and tightens pores.

COSMETIC VINEGARS

Victorian ladies carefully guarded their secret recipes for cosmetic vinegars, for in those days they were often used as a fragrance too (see page 158). Vinegar has an astringent quality and also brings high color to the face. The first time I used vinegar on my face, it became red as a beet, frankly scaring me. But within minutes it calmed down to a nice healthy glow. Later I learned never to use vinegar straight on my face but to dilute it. Following are two special recipes for cosmetic vinegars from the last century. They should be used on oily skin only.

Rose Geranium Vinegar

Mix 1 pint hot water with 1 pint vinegar. Cool, then add 1 teaspoon rose geranium oil. Keep this in a tightly lidded bottle. Use it after cleaning your face to freshen it, tighten the pores, and reduce oiliness.

Red Rose Vinegar

Put 1 ounce dried rose petals (2 tablespoons) in 1 pint white wine vinegar. Let it stand with top on it 2 weeks. Strain, throw away the rose petals, and add 1 cup rose water (page 154). This can be used as is or diluted to remove oil from the skin.

LOTIONS FOR AN ASSORTMENT OF PROBLEMS

Coarse Pore Lotion

This lotion was originated in the nineteenth century expressly to refine coarse pores. Add 1/4 cup glycerin and 1/2 teaspoon borax to 3/4 cup rose water (page 154).

Blend thoroughly. Apply this to the skin and leave it on overnight.

Pimple and Blackhead Lotion

This recipe was given to me by an East Indian friend, Swami Harihardas. Add 1/4 cup lemon juice to 2 tablespoons glycerin. To this add a pinch of nutmeg. Blend well. Keep the mixture in the sun for 7 days. Strain out leaves or any residue which may have fallen into the solution. Use it as a lotion to treat pimples and blackheads.

Swami Harihardas' Wrinkle-Remover

Carefully blend 1 teaspoon rice powder with 1 teaspoon each grapefruit juice, carrot juice, and yogurt. Keep in the sun for 3 hours. Apply to the face overnight to smooth out wrinkles.

Dandelion and Parsley Freckle-Remover

Steep 1 cup dandelions and 1 cup fresh parsley in 1 quart boiling water. Cool the infusion, strain, and apply to freckled areas. The freckles will gradually fade away, they say.

LETTUCE LEAF MOISTURIZER
AND OTHERS

Moisturizers help to plump up the tone and texture of the skin cells by replenishing their lost water. They also maintain the balance of the acid mantle, thus protecting the skin against harsh climatic conditions and bacteria. Normal and oily skins, as well as dry, can benefit from moisturizers and need never fear increased surface oiliness. Moisturizers penetrate the skin's pores, unlike oily creams, which are best used just to clean, since they usually don't go below the surface—although these creams can be culprits in clogging pores. Commercial

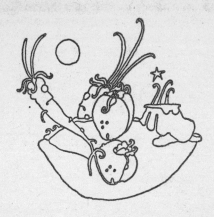

moisturizing lotions have water whipped into them. The natural preparations given here have their own built-in moisturizing qualities. Glycerin, honey, and cucumbers are the oldest moisturizers known to woman. Moisturizers are put on the face last, after all cleaners have been applied. They can be used in the morning, again in the afternoon, at night, and in between all those times. The face always benefits from moisture.

Glycerin and Honey Moisturizer
Mix 9 parts glycerin with 1 part honey. Blend until they are completely mixed. Smooth this all over the face, including the area around the eyes. Keep it on all day and wear it overnight if you wish to keep your skin moist.

Cucumber Moisturizer
Keep half a peeled crisp cucumber in the refrigerator to use as a skin moisturizer. Rub it all over your face and feel its cooling and moisturizing effects, particularly soothing to irritated skin. Cleopatra was supposed to have

used this simple remedy, and our own history tells us that pioneer women used to cut open a cucumber at the end of a day in the fields to freshen their work-parched skins.

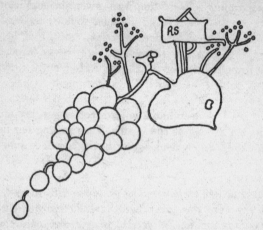

Grape Moisturizer
Keep a bunch of white grapes in the refrigerator so you can pick a few and squeeze them over your face. The juice of white grapes is especially soothing to dry and/or wrinkled skin.

Watermelon Moisturizer
Cut thin slices of watermelon. Lie down with them on your face for 1/2 hour for a moist refresher.

Lettuce Leaf Moisturizer
Boil lettuce leaves for 2 hours in enough distilled water to keep them from scorching in the pan. Cool and use the liquid as is or mix it with yogurt. The French peasants have long used moisturizing lettuce juice to calm angry, irritated skin. In fact, a crisp piece of lettuce can be rubbed directly over the skin to help combat oiliness.

Rainwater
Christine Valmy suggests you "take advantage of a rainy

day by removing all makeup and walking face up for a healthy and stimulating 'rain' massage."

The Nineteenth Century
Englishwoman's Face Bath

This charming information was given in a Victorian beauty book: "Many Englishwomen follow the sensible practice of giving the face a drink. For proof of the efficiency of this, carry to your bathroom a drooping, dying plant. Turn upon it with the rubber spray a shower of cool water. Instantly the fainting plant revives. The Englishwoman closes her eyes, holds her breath, and thrusts her face deep into a bowl of cool water, keeping it submerged as long as she is able. Then raising her head, she breathes deeply and again thrusts her face into the water. She repeats this face drink five or six times, wiping moisture off with a soft cloth. It is amazing to see the response of her complexion to the treatment, transformed from brownish-white parchment, crossed and criss-crossed by the faint etchings that portend wrinkles, to a smooth pink and white silken surface."

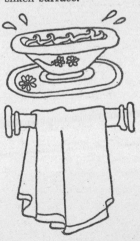

Face Masks and Saunas: Honey, Pine Needles, and Swami Harihardas

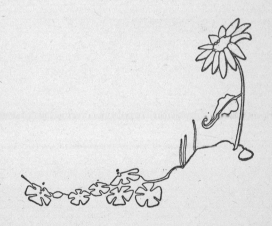

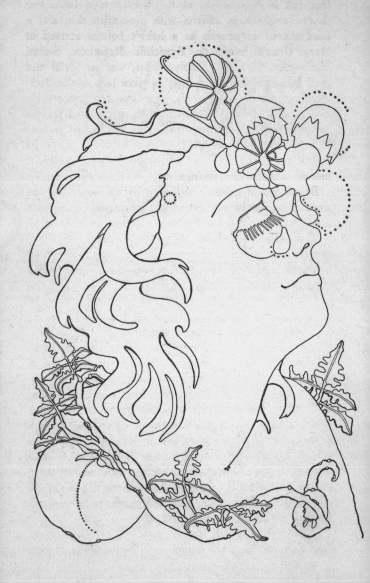

One fall in Woodstock, as the trees turned burnished shades, a vision in saffron with nut-brown skin and a head shaved as smooth as a baby's bottom arrived at Mary Orser's house on Byrdcliffe Mountain. Swami Harihardas, although a holy leader, was so jovial and good humored that it was easy to place him among ordinary mortals. So we sat around Mary's round oak table and chatted, as people do, about the herbs and potions he kept in little silky bags and about the beauty recipes he kept in his head. He told me to sit at his right and he called me Mira; not given to quick name changes, I merely tolerated the gesture.

By afternoon Swami had won us all over, but we women were especially captivated by a mask made with orange and lemon peels, to "make the complexion fair," Swami said. Twelve years studying herbal medicines and other natural preparations made his remedies foolproof, he assured us. The mask was that. We all came out feeling the fairer for it.

Swami's Orange-Lemon Peel Fair Complexion Mask

You need the peels of 1 orange and 1 lemon; the fruits must be organic, according to Swami. This would make the orange green rather than orange. I must now admit to having used orange oranges. Grind the skins fine (sorry, but a grinder of some sort is needed here) and mix them with a tiny amount of water—just enough to make a paste. Apply the paste to your face. Lie in the sun, if it's around, until the paste becomes warm and seeps into your pores; leave it on the skin for 10 to 20 minutes. Wipe off the excess, leaving a coating of natural oils on your skin. The mask will leave your face refreshed, glowing, and waxy smooth.

Masks are as old as the mummies of Egypt. In fact, what

do you think the archaeologists found when they un-
earthed the ruins of Egypt? Beauty shops with perfumery
and cosmetic products and recipes lying around. Recipes
for what? For masks. In truth, all modern products, from
dyes and hair tonics to lipsticks and vitamin creams, had
their counterparts in Egypt of Cleopatra's day.

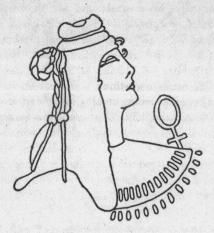

Aunt Myrtle taught me about my first face mask. It
was an egg yolk. It made me feel terrific long before I
cared about being beautiful, and it made my aunt
ageless. To this day I don't know her age, although she's
been around and an adult for as long as I can remember.
She's still blonde, blue-eyed, fair-skinned, and gorgeous.
I remember one time a few years ago both of us looked
in the mirror. I said, "Look, Myrt, neither of us has
wrinkles." This was true, of course, but I was only fifteen,
and she was I don't know what. It must have been the
egg yolk—that and her love of life.

Later in life I visited a facial salon in New York, run
by a famous European cosmetologist. Women in Europe
go to facial salons as often as women here go to beauty

parlors. Luckily, since I was writing a story on the place, I didn't have to pay for the visit. The prices did not then, nor do they now, fit into my budget. But the treatment was exquisite. My face was massaged, masked, steamed, oiled, and ironed. Yes, ironed: A small hand iron, set at a gentle heat, was run smoothly over my oiled skin. This was a special cosmetic iron, mind you, so don't attempt doing it with your General Electric.

It would be nice to go to a facial salon every week. I'm not knocking it, price and all. But since it's out of range of most of our change purses, do the same thing at home. Practically everything that went on in that salon, save for the pink smocks and the lovely carpet, can be substituted for. Make yourself a smock if you need the ambience. I don't need that, but the iron was something else. I know how to imitate it. Someone told me. With a spoon. Yes. Put warm unctuous oil—almond is fine—on your face. Warm up a tablespoon, not so hot that it will hurt you, but warm. Then run the back of the spoon over your oiled face. Iron and iron and iron.

Facial massages, masks, saunas, and exercises are all given in this chapter. The oils and the creams you learned about in the last one.

MASSAGE . . .

The purpose of a facial massage is to stimulate circulation and to oil and smooth out wrinkles. A thick, unctuous oil or cream is used for facial massaging. Apply the oil to your skin 20 minutes before the massage begins. Wrap your hair in a towel to keep it off your face and neck.

Begin at the neck. It should be massaged with the

length of the fingers, moving in an upward motion from chest and shoulders to chin. On the face, the fingertips alone are used. The motion is upward and rotating. It's good to remember to use this upward movement whenever you're drying your face or applying creams and lotions.

A young face can be stimulated with a fairly hearty massage, whereas older skin requires a gentler hand. The purpose is to stimulate rather than to stretch the skin. For mature skins a tapping, vibrating movement with the tips of the fingers give the skin sufficient stimulation.

Coconut Oil Massage Cream

Melt 1/4 cup white wax or beeswax, 2 tablespoons lanolin, and 1/4 cup coconut oil in an enamel or glass double boiler. Beat in rose water (page 154) a little at a time until the desired consistency is achieved. When the mixture is nearly cool, stir in a few drops of your favorite essential oil for fragrance. Refrigerate.

. . . AND MASK

Massaging before a mask is applied makes pores more receptive to the mask. The face must also be impeccably clean before the mask is applied.

Masks serve so many purposes that it's surprising that many women neglect to use them. They nourish the skin. They have astringent powers. Yeast, a popular mask ingredient rich in the B vitamins (known to keep skin smooth and regulate secretions), is a powerful astringent for oily skins, although it's used for other types too.

Once on the face, a mask begins to pull and tighten and tone skin. The usual time to leave it on the face is 10 to 20 minutes, although a strongly astringent mask, which dries like concrete, may be uncomfortable if left for longer than 5 minutes. Because of the tightening quality of masks, the tender areas around the eyes should be left free of the application. In fact, the eye area could be covered with compresses while the mask is taking effect.

Some masks—avocado, for example—soften and moisturize. Often the residue is merely wiped off, leaving a coating of the vegetable's or fruit's natural oils. Most masks, however, are rinsed off with warm water, with an additional splash of cold following to increase the circulatory performance.

All masks, some more than others, have a deep pore-cleaning action. One of the added benefits of a mask is that the ingredients often force you to be in repose, so two things are accomplished: a beauty treatment and a beauty rest.

NORMAL SKIN MASKS

Honey and Lemon Mask

Mix 1 tablespoon slightly warmed honey with 1 teaspoon lemon juice. Carefully blend the ingredients. Apply this to your face. Leave the mixture on for 1/2 hour or even longer. This has a special moisturizing effect on the skin. It's good for dry skin too. (Pineapple juice can be substituted for the lemon when you want a change.)

Yogurt, Mint, and Fuller's Earth Mask

Mix 1 teaspoon peppermint extract with 1 tablespoon water. Add enough yogurt and fuller's earth (available at drugstores) in equal parts to make a paste. Apply the mask to the skin and leave it on 10 to 15 minutes. Rinse it off with warm water, then a dash of cold. The mint gives the skin a menthol feeling.

Wheat Germ——Honey Mask

Combine 1 tablespoon honey with 1 tablespoon dry wheat germ. Apply this liberally to your face. Leave it on for 20 minutes or until your face feels tingly. Remove it with warm water, then a pat of icy cold. This serves to cleanse, stimulate, and refresh the face.

Honey-Apple Mask

Cut an apple into small pieces and place it in a bowl. Mash it with a fork until it is a pulp. Add an approximate equal amount of honey to the apple pulp and then mix the two thoroughly together. Apply this to your face for 10 to 15 minutes. Rinse it off with warm water, followed by cold. This mask leaves your face refreshed, moist, and glowing.

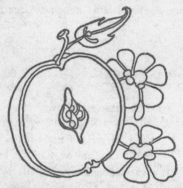

Egg White Mask

This is a simple but extremely effective mask. Crack open an egg. Separate the white from the yolk and apply the white to your face. Leave it on for about 20 minutes. Rinse it off with warm water followed by a splash of cold. This mask can be used 2 or 3 times a week, but only once if your face tends to be dry. It removes impurities from the pores and leaves your face soft, smooth, and glowing. This mask also works wonders when your face is tired and puffy. They also say it's good for a hangover.

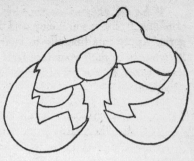

DRY SKIN MASKS

Yeast and Wheat Germ Oil Mask

Combine 1 tablespoon powdered brewer's yeast with 1/2 teaspoon wheat germ oil. This should make a paste. If it's not the consistency you like, add more oil. Leave it on your face for 10 to 15 minutes, then wash it off with warm water. (Cold water contracts the pores, and as the purpose here is to stimulate the skin's oil to rise to the surface, best to avoid it.) Apply some of the oil to your face before going to bed. This mask stimulates the production of natural oils. When your face is very dry, use it twice a week.

Tomato Mask

Slice a ripe tomato as thin as possible. Apply the slices to your face, then lie down and close your eyes for 10 to 15 minutes. Let the juices seep into your skin. After the 10 to 15 minutes are up, use a slice to rub the juices further into the skin. Do this over the sink, as it is messy. The tomato works in effect like a face peel, removing all dead, dry skin and leaving your face soft, glossy, and smooth. Rub off the excess tomato, leaving the residue on your skin. The mild natural acidity of the tomato restores the acid mantle balance of the skin.

Avocado Mask

Mash an avocado with some vegetable oil until it is as

creamy as it can get. Rub it into your skin. Let it remain on your face while you nap for 10 to 15 minutes. Rinse it off with warm water or rub off the excess, leaving some of the oil on your face. The natural oil of the avocado gives a smooth glow to your face.

Egg-Honey Rose Water Mask

Combine 1 egg yolk and 2 tablespoons egg white with 1 tablespoon honey and 1 teaspoon rose water (page 154). Beat this together with a fork. Apply it to your face. Let it dry for 10 to 15 minutes, then remove it with warm water. Apply a lubricant like almond oil after removing the mask. This mask is helpful when the skin is not only dry but also showing a tendency to wrinkle.

Banana Mask

Mash 1 ripe banana and rub it lavishly into your face. Leave it on for 15 to 20 minutes, napping if you wish. Rinse it off with warm water or merely remove the residue, leaving a thin coat of oil on your face. The natural banana oils penetrate the skin, relieving dryness.

Olive Oil Mask

Soak cotton pads in warm olive oil. Have a hot towel ready. Cover your face with the pads. Place the towel over your face so that the heat penetrates the oil-saturated pads and then the skin. Keep the towel on your face until it's cool. Redo the process if your face is extremely dry. Don't disturb the coating of oil left after the hot towel treatment. This couldn't be better for restoring oil to a parched face.

OILY SKIN MASKS

Oatmeal and Milk Mask

Mix oatmeal with milk to make a paste, then spread it on your face and leave it there for 10 to 15 minutes. Rinse it off with warm water; splash on cold. Apply a freshener

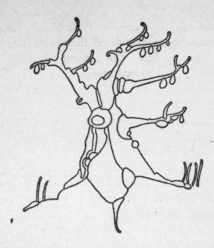

if you wish. This miracle skin food, oatmeal, effective on all parts of the body, makes a splendid mask for removing excess oil from the skin.

Oatmeal with Honey or Egg Mask

Oatmeal mixed with honey or egg to make a paste is effective as a mask when skin suffers from blackheads, as well as excess oiliness.

Honey and Dry Milk Mask

Mix 1 teaspoon powdered skim milk with 1/2 teaspoon honey. Beat this mixture with an egg white until the ingredients are thoroughly blended. Apply it thickly to your face. Let it remain for 15 to 20 minutes. Remove it with warm water, followed by a splash of cold. This unclogs pores and combats excess oiliness.

Brewer's Yeast Mask

Mix 1 tablespoon powdered brewer's yeast with a small amount of witch hazel—just enough to make a paste. Leave this on your face; it will harden like clay. Rinse it off with warm water, then with cold. Due to its severe astringent power, this mask leaves even the oiliest skin quite dry. You may want to follow it with a skin lubricant. The mask clears away oiliness and penetrates pores to remove blackheads.

Yeast Cake Mask

This mask is even more astringent than the preceding one; it hardens on your face like concrete. Although the noun "concrete" sounds formidable, the mask is good for you. Add enough water to 1 yeast cake to turn it into a paste. Apply this to your face. Leave it on for 15 to 20 minutes or for as long as you can take it. Remove it with warm water, then splash on some cold. Apply a mild skin moisturizer—a lettuce or grape one (see page 58). This mask does a fine job when your skin is overly oily and afflicted with blackheads.

Egg—Bicarbonate of Soda—Lemon Mask

Drop a pinch of bicarbonate of soda into 1 beaten egg yolk. Add 12 drops lemon juice. Mix well. Apply this to your face. Leave it on for 10 to 15 minutes. Remove it with warm water, then rinse with cold. Apply a mild freshener. This removes excess oil.

Barley Flour, Honey, and Egg Mask

This Victorian face mask contains all kinds of good things to make it applicable today. Mix 6 tablespoons barley flour with 2 tablespoons honey and 1 teaspoon egg white to form a paste. Leave this on your face for 10 to 15 minutes. Remove it with warm water, followed by cold. This mask stimulates circulation and removes excess oil and impurities.

FACIAL SAUNAS

A facial sauna, like a mask, unclogs pores. It's possible to have a facial mask and subsequently a sauna if the pores still need work; however, when skin is sensitive, it's best to go easy. Alternate—a mask every few days, a sauna in between.

Many things can be called facial saunas; in fact, the term applies to anything that steams the face. A hot towel does this. The steam from water brought to a boil in a pan (with the heat turned off when you're ready to use it) does this. Or water, with a few menthol and purgative ingredients added to it, can be boiled, then placed in the bathroom sink. With a towel placed over your head and the sink, forming a tent to capture the mist, you steam your face. Then there are faily inexpensive commercial saunas, scientifically controlled for sensitive skins to reach a gentle 118 degrees. Whatever the sauna method used, the result is the same: As the skin perspires, oil and makeup loosen, pores unplug. Clean skin!

Pine and Chamomile Sauna

When I am in Vermont, I gather pine needles right from the trees and chamomile, growing wild, right from the ground. A handful of each is put in a quart pan of water that has been brought to a boil. A few teaspoons of camphor are added. Then the mixture is poured into the bathroom sink. I put a towel around my head to form a tent so steam won't escape, never letting the hot water touch my skin. Sometimes it gets quite hot, but I

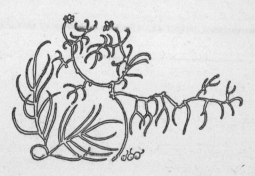

hold my face in the steam as long as I can take it. Often I have to come out from under the tent for a second and then go under again. But it's amazing how the pores do open up and clean themselves out.

Rosemary Sauna

Steep a handful of the herb rosemary in water that has been brought to a boil. To steam your face use the vapors from the pot or remove the mixture to the bathroom basin. Large pores are minimized, blackheads removed. This is great for teen-age (or, for that matter, adult) acne.

Clove and Eucalyptus Oil Sauna

Combine 1 tablespoon oil of cloves with 1 tablespoon oil of eucalyptus in a quart of fast-boiling water. Use this to steam your face. This sauna, due to the oily consistency of the ingredients, is good for dry skins, which might be sensitive to other types.

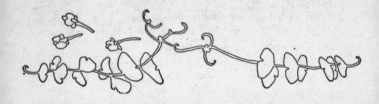

EXERCISES FOR FACE AND NECK

Now that you're involved in your own facial salon, throw in a few exercises. There are fifty-five muscles in the face which need constant strenghtening so that in later years they don't give way on you. Funny, but women will spend time on stomach exercises and forget the face and neck, the parts that show first and clearest.

Start early enough to train these muscles, and later they won't sag or go flabby. A few minutes of minimum effort can actually retard lines and flab. Before beginning the following exercises, apply a lubricating cream or oil so that there's no possible way your face will retain the wrinkles you make when you perform these facial acrobatics.

The first face exercise begins early in the morning when you yawn. Open your mouth wide and give a special go at it. Jut out your bottom jaw. Let it drop. Then with restraint, pulling all the neck muscles with it, pull the jaw and bottom row of teeth up over your upper lip. This exercise helps to eliminate a double chin.

Next, when you look in the mirror and hate the sight of yourself—or love it; I don't know—make faces to waken up a slack expression and promote stimulation. Pop your eyes out. Stick your tongue out until the jaw and neck muscles feel the pull. Pull your nose and move it around clockwise. Gather your hair back in one hand and pull up, lifting your neck out of its slump.

Purse your lips so they stick out as far as possible. In this position move them from right to left and back to center. Repeat. This tightens up neck muscles and keeps small lines from forming around the mouth.

Try "blowing bubble gum" as another exercise to help eliminate lines around the mouth.

Make big eyes, opening them as wide as possible. Then close them very tight. Repeat this several times to keep your eyelids from becoming flabby.

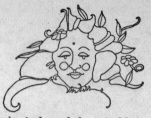

TO SUM IT UP

"If it be true that 'the face is the index of the mind,' the recipe for a beautiful face must be something that reaches the soul. What can be done for a human face that has a sluggish, sullen, arrogant, angry mind looking out of every feature? An habitually ill-natured, discontented mind ploughs the face with inevitable marks of its own vices. However bright its complexion, no such face can ever become really beautiful." So said the beautiful, inimitable Lola Montez in 1853.

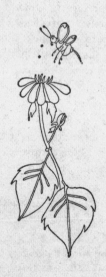

Hair:
Chamomile,
Peanut Flour,
and
St. Paul's Prejudice

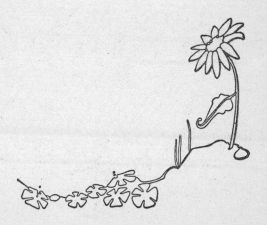

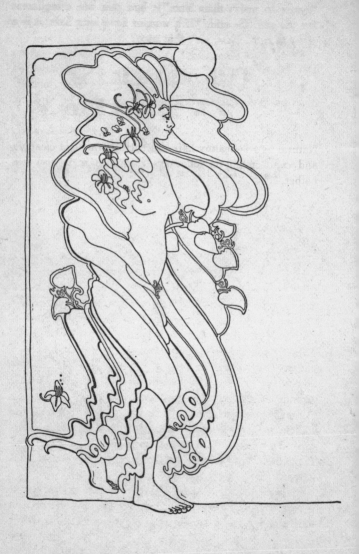

St. Paul, that great old male chauvinist who warned men to stay away from women (although adding that it was "better to marry than burn"), had this one compliment for our sex: He said, "If a woman have long hair, it is a glory to her." Now, isn't that nice?

These days when earth mothers are in flower, we *are* glorying in long hair, finally letting it go the way God meant it to be. No bleaching, dyeing, crimping, marcelling, permanenting, straightening, curling, or kinking, not for most of us. Straight hair grows two to three feet long; curly heads ruffle up Pre-Raphaelite-like. Natural hair is healthy hair if a correct course of cleaning and conditioning is followed. Natural hair is also less bother.

HAIRY TALES

One Christmas I saw a doll that grows hair. Right—you turn a knob, and the hair moves upward and outward from the scalp. Horrible doll, but a graphic example: For the most part, we treat our hair as though it began at the hairline, forgetting growth begins within the scalp.

Like skin, the scalp has pores, about a thousand to a square inch. The hair "pores" are called follicles. Hair grows out of the follicles, about 100,000 to 140,000 strands' worth to the average head.

Small hair cells form in a tiny white bulb at the follicle root, one tenth of an inch below the scalp's surface. These cells stick to and overlap one another until they push out of the follicle, becoming longer and longer.

Hair grows about half an inch a month, six inches in a year. By the time a person reaches the age of fifty, the hair could reach a length of twenty-five feet and weigh over sixteen pounds except for this: The weight of each hair would loosen the support of the muscles that grip the root, and the hair would probably fall out. These muscles usually relax their grip on hair when it reaches a length of two to three feet. Then hairs fall out, but one by one, and new ones replace them.

It's unlikely all your hair would ever fall out at once unless severe damage was done that weakened every follicle muscle at one time. Massaging the scalp insures that this will probably never happen.

Whether hair and scalp are oily or dry is determined by each follicle's oil gland. Daily that gland produces oil, which is distributed by the hairbrush or massage and every few days washed away by shampooing and rinsing to make room for more natural oil. When hair and head are not kept clean, excess oil piles up and cakes on the scalp. Fresh oils can't reach the hair and scalp to lubricate them. There is no acid mantle to protect them. One theory is that the accumulation of excess oil and dirt produces a flaky dandruff-like residue which eventually damages the hair follicles. Hair begins to fall out. Everything is a mess.

Hair and scalp need external treatment. They are affected by dirt, by their own oils, by dandruff, by sun and harsh weather, which fade and bleach color. On the other hand, they are also affected by massage, shampooing, conditioning, and rinses, all positive things that brighten and restore hair and scalp.

MASSAGE

Massage loosens up tight scalps, and at the same time, dirt, oil, bacteria, and dandruff that have gathered there. Massage stimulates circulation of blood to the scalp, normalizes the production of oil glands, improves the growth and luster of the hair. It also helps to keep you from going bald.

There are two ways to massage hair and scalp: with a brush and with your hands. Usually hair, unless fine, brittle, overbleached, or overly oily, should be brushed every day with a brush with stiff natural bristles, never harsh nylon or synthetic ones. Brush hair upward or downward (if you're hanging your head over) and forward, until the scalp tingles, distributing natural oils throughout. Actual clinically termed dandruff—as opposed to the dandruff-like substance that forms on the scalp from excess dirt and oil—is thought to be caused by a contagious germ, so keep your brush to yourself. Rub bran in the brush bristles between brushings, then comb out excess. At week's end dip the brush into 3 teaspoonfuls ammonia in 1/2 a mixing-size bowl of warm water to completely remove grease and dirt.

Normal scalps should be massaged once a week; with hair loss or dandruff present, three or four times is not too much. To massage the scalp place the fingers of each hand on the crown of the head, the thumbs at the temples; rotate them all at once, moving the fingers all over the head.

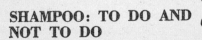

SHAMPOO: TO DO AND NOT TO DO

Shampoo as often as your hair and scalp need it. This could be every day if they're very oily, the climate's sticky and hot, you work in a boiler room, or you live in a city like New York, where pollution is a way of life.

Avoid detergent shampoos. Use shampoos based on castile soap or natural oils. I know of two commercial shampoos that are castile-based: Johnson's Baby Shampoo and Breck Shampoo. Non-detergent shampoos are usually sold at health food stores.

My favorite shampoo is Dr. Bronner's Peppermint-Oil Soap (100% natural coconut, peppermint oil, and pure castile soap), available at health food stores. I add rosemary, my favorite herb, to it. Dr. Bronner's makes good reading too: The plastic bottle's label claims the soap washes everything from your teeth to your car. It also has words of religious and philosophic uplift which sound something like the ranting that goes on in Bryant Park, New York, but as a shampoo Dr. Bronner's is unsurpassed.

HOW TO SHAMPOO

After brushing and massaging your hair and scalp, wet them thoroughly with warm water and apply shampoo. Starting at your forehead, lather up the shampoo as you scrub backward, massaging your scalp all the while. When hair and scalp have been well shampooed, rinse with warm water. Soap, massage, and rinse two or three times until your hair squeaks when you pull a strand between your fingers.

As with skin pores, warm water expands hair follicles, cold water contracts. Common sense says that the last rinse for dry hair is warm, and for oily, cold. The rinse can be plain water, vinegar, or one of the prepared rinses coming up.

Dry your hair thoroughly, in the sun if possible, rubbing each strand with your fingers to help the process.

Don't use a brush until your hair is completely dry, as wet strands are more susceptible to breakage.

Years ago it was fashionable to dry each strand of hair with a piece of silk to give it literally a silky sheen. It's a wonderful way to enhance your feelings of self-worth, as to do this requires a great deal of time expended on yourself.

Homemade Castile Shampoo

Shave a bar of pure castile soap into a pot of water simmering on the stove. (Experiment to find the exact consistency you like, since the recipe can vary anywhere from 1 bar castile soap to 1 pint water all the way to 1/2 bar to 2 quarts.) Dissolve the soap over a slow flame. Rainwater is terrific to use, but a pinch of borax will also soften water.

Chamomile Shampoo

Steep 1 cup chamomile blossoms (or rosemary) in 1 quart boiling water. Strain off the liquid and simmer it over low heat, slowly adding 2 tablespoons castile soap shavings. Stir until the soap dissolves. Chamomile is for blondes, rosemary for darker hair; each brings out natural highlights.

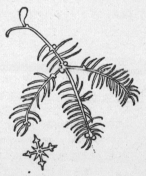

Pine Tar Dandruff Shampoo

Use this to shampoo oily dark hair only. Dissolve 1 bar

castile soap in 1 pint hot water. Add 1 tablespoon oil of pine tar or oil of birch tar and 2 tablespoonfuls alcohol. Shampoo into the hair to remove dandruff. Rinse several times.

Green Soap Dandruff Shampoo

Add 1 teaspoon tincture of green soap to 2 beaten egg whites and 10 drops cologne. Use this shampoo to remove dandruff. Rinse thoroughly.

Wheat Bran Dry Shampoo

Because of illness or mere lack of time, a dry shampoo is sometimes necessary. Wheat bran, cornmeal, or powered orris root (used separately or combined in equal parts) sprinkled on the hair with a salt shaker, then carefully brushed through, a few strands at a time, removes oil and dirt; so does a hairbrush covered with an old nylon stocking.

Dry shampoos will cake in the hair after repeated applications, so it's advisable to use them only once or twice between regular shampoos. They may also leave white flakes in red hair, so a flame-haired friend of mine suggests adding a little cinnamon to the mixture.

HERBAL HAIR CONDITIONERS AND OTHERS

Hair conditioners are essential for preserving and correcting the condition of the scalp and hair, overcoming disorders like dandruff and hair loss and stimulating the bloodstream so it nourishes the scalp. Herbal conditioners can be used after washing hair. Messier treatments that use eggs or castor oil should be applied to clean hair and followed by another shampoo and rinse.

Swami's Peanut Conditioner

In India women use this conditioner to restore oils that

have been dried out by the sun. Use equal amounts peanut flour (can be found at health food stores), lemon juice, and yogurt. Scrub the mixture into the hair and wash it out with Dr. Bronner's or with castile shampoo and warm water. Follow up with a vinegar rinse for a terrific protein conditioning.

Note: If peanut flour is not available, ask the proprietor of a health food store to grind up peanuts for you.

Herbal Mixture Treatment

Claire Loewenfeld and Phillipa Back have written a very fine book, *Herbs, Health & Cookery*, in which they give an excellent hair rinse utilizing several herbs, both household ones—lime flowers, chamomile, fennel, sage, and rosemary—and ones that grow wild—nettles, horsetails, and yarrow. For light hair, the lime flowers, chamomile, and fennel are mixed in larger equal parts, the others in smaller equal parts. For dark hair, the same recipe is used, except that rosemary becomes a larger

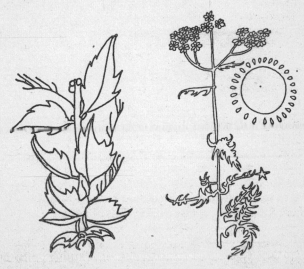

part and chamomile is reduced to a smaller one. This
special herbal mixture, say Loewenfeld and Back, "has
a stimulating effect on the glands and tissues of the scalp
and stimulates growth and healthy development of the
hair." This and all herbal mixtures must be newly prepared before each application.

Nettle Dandruff Tonic

Steep 1 teaspoon nettles in 1 cup vinegar that has been
brought to a boil. Dip the fingers into the mixture and
apply to the scalp, thoroughly massaging it in. Rinse it
out. This cures dandruff. Nettles steeped in water rather
than in vinegar work to liven up the color of dull, faded
hair; with water as the base, this nettle tea need not be
rinsed out.

Rosemary, Burdock, Sage, and Thyme Dandruff Tonic

Mix 1 teaspoon each rosemary, grated burdock root,
sage, and thyme. Steep the herbs in 1 pint boiling water,
then strain the liquid through cheesecloth. Rub part of
the mixture into the scalp and pour the rest through the
hair to remove dandruff.

Mint Dandruff Tonic

Add 1 cup mint leaves (fresh if available) to 1 cup white
vinegar and 2 cups water. Boil this together slowly for
5 to 10 minutes. Strain it. Cool liquid. Rub the solution
into the scalp to remove dandruff. Rinse well.

Egg White–Lemon Dry Scalp Treatment

Whip up the whites of 2 eggs with the strained juice of
2 lemons. Rub the mixture lavishly into the scalp with
the fingertips to remove flaky, itchy residue and restore
natural oils.

Mayonnaise Split End Conditioner

Lisa Kosman, sales manager of The Good Earth, a New
York health food store, applies 2 tablespoons mayonnaise
to her scalp after shampooing her waist-length red hair.
She works the mayonnaise through the length of her hair,

leaving it on 1 hour to condition split ends. Then she rinses it out. Mayonnaise contains egg (protein and lecithin), vinegar (acid), and vegetable oil. But heed this: If your hair is shorter and finer than Miss Kosman's, use less mayonnaise. I followed her directions verbatim, and my shorter, finer hair became quite oily, needing several shampoos and rinses. Later I used a mere teaspoon of mayonnaise and found it worked well on my split ends.

Yogurt–Lemon Rind Bleached Hair Conditioner

Combine equal amounts yogurt and grated lemon rind (1 teaspoon each for shorter hair, more for longer). Generously rub this into the scalp, pulling it through the hair. The yogurt, with its natural concentrated protein, nourishs dry, sun- or chemical-bleached hair; the lemon rind adds natural oils and luster.

Whole Egg Conditioner for Dull, Brittle Hair

Beat 2 eggs until fluffy. Work them carefully into clean hair. Leave this on for 1/2 hour or more. Rinse it out with warm water, followed by a shampoo, a vinegar rinse, and more warm water to leave hair healthy and shining.

Egg Yolk–Yogurt Conditioner for Dull, Brittle Hair

Beat 1 egg yolk until fluffy. To it add 1/2 cup yogurt and beat again until thoroughly mixed. Comb this mixture through clean hair. Leave it on for 10 minutes, then rinse thoroughly with warm water. Follow up with a vinegar rinse and more warm water. This leaves the hair soft and lustrous.

Olive Oil Conditioner for Dry, Brittle Hair

My friend Jean Conlon, who once labored through a book with me (*Beauty Is No Big Deal*, 1971), swears by this conditioner, which, in fact, we mentioned in that book. Rub olive oil into the scalp and then comb it through the rest of the hair. Wrap the head with terry towels so the oil can penetrate the hair follicles. Four steaming-hot towels applied over 1 hour's time are not too many. Shampoo well and rinse with vinegar. Follow with warm water. Caution: This treatment is quite oily and so should be used but once a month and then only on thick, dry hair.

Castor Oil Conditioner for Dry, Brittle Hair

According to Linda Clark in *Secrets of Health and Beauty*, castor oil makes hair 9.2 percent stronger (the next best strengthener is liquid lanolin, at 2.4 percent). Rub the castor oil liberally into the scalp. Follow with the 4-towel treatment described in the preceding recipe. This is excellent for dry, brittle hair. A folk remedy for falling hair mentioned by Deborah Rutledge in *Natural Beauty Secrets* uses castor oil on the hair one day, followed by white iodine the next. This pattern is followed for four days. Apply just enough castor oil to massage the scalp; too much is messy. On the fourth day more oil can be used, followed by the "4-towel treatment." Shampoo well and rinse.

Egg Yolk–Baking Soda Oily-Hair Conditioner

Dissolve 1 teaspoon bicarbonate of soda in 1 pint warm water. Into this blend 2 well-beaten eggs. Rub part of this into the scalp. Pour the rest over the hair and comb it through. Shampoo and rinse. This is a nineteenth century remedy for reducing oiliness.

Egg–Rum–Rose Water Hair-Brightening Treatment

Beat 4 egg whites to a froth. Rub them thoroughly into scalp and leave them to dry. Wash them out and rinse with equal parts rum and rose water (see page 154). The author of the nineteenth century beauty book where this was found claims this to be "one of the best cleansers and brighteners of the hair that was ever used."

A FRAGRANT GERANIUM RINSE
AND OTHERS

As a lotion or astringent follows a face-cleaning, a rinse follows a hair-washing to cut through dust, dirt, excess oil, and film left over after shampooing. Rinses soften hair, giving it a fluffy finish. Sometimes these preparations strengthen the hair shaft. When they are citric or acidic rinses, the acid mantle is restored. And often the natural coloring ingredient in the rinse is reflected in the shade of your hair.

Lemon Rinse for Oily Blonde Hair

Lemon has a light bleaching quality, making it a good rinse for blondes, both natural and bleached (with the latter, it separates hair strands, which tend to be porous and so cling together). Add the strained juice of 3 lemons to 1 pint water. Pour this through the hair several times to brighten it. When hair is exceptionally oily, 1 teaspoonful salt may be added to the rinse.

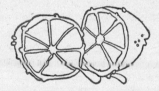

Chamomile Rinse for Born Blondes

Chamomile grows wild in Vermont, where I live part of the year. We pick it to make teas, to steam our faces, and if we are blonde, to rinse our hair. I'm not blonde, but my friend Caroline is. This is the rinse she uses: Steep 1/4 cup chamomile flowers in 1 quart boiling water. Strain off the liquid and cool it. Use it as a final rinse to brighten blonde hair. Do not rinse it off. This herb adds strength to the hair and acts as a tonic for the scalp.

Chamomile-Vinegar Rinse for Bleached Blondes

The same chamomile rinse Caroline uses brightens bleached hair if 1 teaspoon vinegar is added to restore the acid mantle, separate hairs, and remove the spongy, sticky feeling that often occurs when hair is bleached.

Chamomile-Henna Rinse for Light Brown Hair

Chamomile also brightens light brown hair. An addition of 1 tablespoon henna added to the chamomile rinse above will give this hair color red highlights.

Chamomile–French Bluing Rinse for Gray or Light Brown Hair

Use the chamomile rinse recipe above with a mere dash of bluing added to the rinse water—just enough to turn it light blue. Use bluing alone when the hair is all gray or white, but keep the rinse water a pale blue shade. This removes all tones of yellow and makes the gray shade more even. Rinse out the bluing with clear water so only a slight bit remains on the hair. Use a little rubbing alcohol to remove any bluing from the face. As these days bluing has generally been added to powdered detergents, it may be difficult to find if sold separately; if so, special order it through your grocer or druggist.

Rosemary Rinse for Brunette Hair

Rosemary is my favorite herb for face and hair. I like its scent too. Following a lathering with Dr. Bronner's Peppermint-Oil Soap, I rinse with an infusion of rosemary made this way: Steep 2 tablespoons rosemary in 1 pint boiling water. Strain off liquid. Let it stand until cold. Rinse the hair with it to fluff it up and bring out natural highlights. Do not rinse it out.

Cider Vinegar Rinse for Brunette Hair

Add 2 tablespoons vinegar to 1 quart water. Pour this

through the hair several times. Rinse it out to remove any vinegar odor. This softens dark hair and gives it luster. A vinegar rinse is also good for dark hair that's been dyed, since it restores the acid mantle and separates strands of hair that may be sticky and porous.

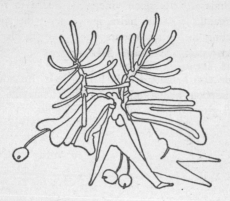

Rosemary—Jamaica Rum Rinse for Brunette Hair

This was a favorite recipe around the time of the Civil War. Here is how it went: Steep 1/4 cup rosemary in 1 pint just-boiled water. Cover this until it's cool. Strain off liquid. Add 5 tablespoons Jamaica rum to the mixture. Pour the rinse through the hair to give it radiance.

Sage Tea Hair-Darkening Rinse

A sage tea rinse is prepared the same way as you would prepare ordinary tea. The tea can temporarily darken any hair color several shades, depending upon its strength. To darken hair about one shade steep a handful of sage in 1 quart boiling water. Steam off liquid. Cool this and pour it over the hair. Leave it on 10 to 20 minutes and rinse it out with clear water. Like any hair rinse, this gives a temporary tinge of color. It usually lasts from one shampoo to the next. I haven't tried this, so you're on your own.

Henna Rinse for Redheads

The ancient Egyptians discovered that the leaves of the henna plant could be used as a hair color. Henna has been serving that purpose ever since, but just now it's hard to get in some places. You may have to ask your druggist to special order it for you. This is how a henna rinse is made: Steep (never boil) 1 cup dry henna leaves in enough boiling water to cover for about 10 minutes. Strain off the liquid. While it's still warm, pour the rinse through the hair until the desired shade is achieved. As the porous ends of the hair absorb henna more quickly than the roots, apply the liquid with a cotton swab to the roots first, giving them a head start. This rinse brightens natural auburn hair. For a golden-red shade add 1 teaspoon chamomile. Henna is a natural coloring agent that also adds strength to the hair.

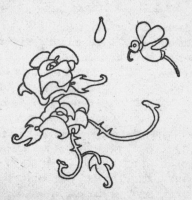

A Fragrant Geranium Rinse

Pick a handful of geraniums and their leaves. Let them steep in 1 quart water that has just been brought to a boil. Strain off the liquid and pour it over the hair. Don't rinse it out. This gives luster and a lovely natural fragrance to the hair. It can be used on all hair colors except perhaps blonde; as blonde hair seems to be very susceptible to color changes, I'd stick with lemon and chamomile.

A Fragrant Honey Rinse

Honey was the name given to this fashionable rinse used by nineteenth century European ladies, although not a trace of the sweet substance is found in the recipe.

> 1 teaspoon essence of ambergris
> 1 teaspoon essence of musk
> 2 teaspoons essence of bergamot
> 1 teaspoon oil of clove
> 1/2 cup orange flower water
> 10 tablespoons alcohol (70%)
> 1/2 cup distilled water

Real ambergris and musk are very expensive, so it's best to buy the synthetic varieties. If you're religiously against synthetics, remember that these essences are from rare animals, so it's ecologically sound not to buy the real things. The ingredients are mixed together, left about 14 days so that the fragrance will take, and then filtered through porous paper and bottled. This makes a good hair wash with an excellent perfume. Alcohol is drying, though, so don't use this rinse on dry, brittle hair.

SETTING LOTIONS

These days many women don't set their hair, but if you do, here are setting lotions to add body to hair and make it manageable.

Gelatin Dessert Setting Lotion

Prepare lemon- or lime-flavored gelatin dessert according to package directions. The liquid gelatin (a source of natural protein), with the addition of the flavoring (citric acid), makes a good setting lotion to give body to hair.

Beer-Lemon Setting Lotion

Mix 1 cup stale beer with 2 tablespoons strained lemon juice. Comb this through the hair after shampooing. It's an excellent setting lotion that makes hair manageable.

Skim Milk Setting Lotion

Stir 6 tablespoons powdered skim milk into 1-1/2 cups water to make it liquid. Comb this through the hair before setting it to make it soft and manageable. For very dry hair substitute 1 cup regular whole milk for the skim milk.

Egg White Setting Lotion

Use 1 part egg white to 2 parts water to give body to hair and make it soft and manageable.

AND FINALLY . . .

For a Hairy Problem

When gum or candy sticks in hair, freeze it out with an ice cube.

These are only a few of many natural hair preparations, the most sensible and least bothersome ones, I think. To give a few examples of stranger ones: In Pericles' time, when blondes were at the height of fashion, Greeks rubbed their hair with goat's fat, beech ashes, and yellow flowers to turn their dark hair golden. A quicker but hardly palatable way to lighten hair was to eat crow's liver or swallow's dung. Cleopatra used bear's grease or natural lanolin to make her hair grow—okay if you can find a bear and then face sacrificing him for a little grease. People were as silly about their cosmetics in ancient times as we are today.

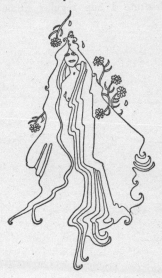

Hands and Nails:
Cornmeal,
Myrrh,
and
Sarah Bernhardt

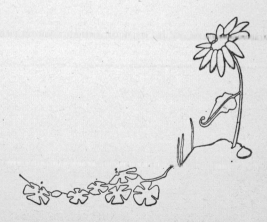

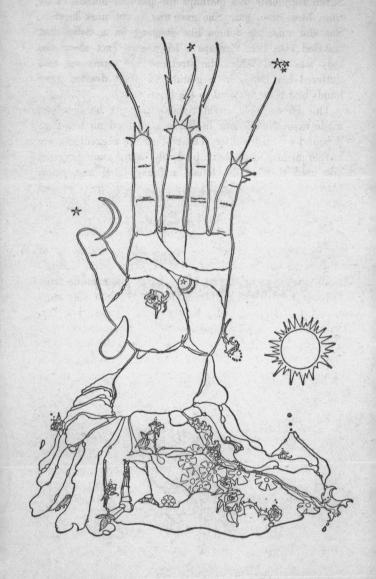

Sarah Bernhardt was perhaps the greatest actress of all time. More than that: She gave rise to the most legends. She did amazing things like sleeping in a coffin that traveled with her. Perhaps a less-known fact about the lady was this: When she stretched her arms out and fluttered her hands in a gesture of great drama, those hands had been buttered to the fingertips.

This is true. The great Sarah's favorite hand lotion, made expressly for her in Paris, contained no less than a pound of fresh butter. The rest of the ingredients are lost to history, but there probably were some fragrant oils used to give the lotion a fancy label and price. Madame could have easily gone to the refrigerator and applied the butter directly, as you can do. Butter contains animal fat; margarine, vegetable oil; both are good lubricants for the hands.

The chief enemies of the hands are too much water and exposure to cold weather. A nineteenth century beauty recommended that ladies carry their muffs from October to April—sensible advice then but a silly solution for girls today who barely wear clothes. The best hand protection for young women, who nowadays consider even wearing cotton or kid gloves an antirevolutionary act, is to wear rubber ones when washing dishes. Water does dehydrate skin and weaken nails, no matter

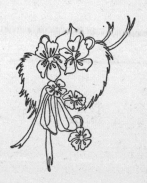

how much the soap companies claim it's their competitors' products that do it. Granted, many girls are too independent even to wear rubber gloves; so if you don't carry a muff or wear cotton or kid or even rubber gloves, keep a bottle of hand lotion next to the kitchen sink to restore skin oils after washing a batch of dishes—that, or go to the refrigerator and take out the butter.

FEEDING CORNMEAL TO YOUR HANDS

Simple cornmeal can be used to remove all manner of dirt, oil, and grease. It is soothing to rough, reddened hands that are sensitive to regular soap. It also makes a good bleaching solution to remove, at least partially, freckles and dark spots from the hands.

Cornmeal Cleaner
Place 1 cup cornmeal and 1/2 cup finely shaved castile soap in a glass jar. Shake and stir well. Wet the hands and apply the mixture to wash them. This is great for dirty, grimy hands that are sensitive to harsh soaps.

Cornmeal Bleaching Paste
Combine 3 parts cornmeal and 2 parts lemon juice, adding enough rose water (see page 154) to make a paste. This mixture is said to bleach freckles and dark spots from hands.

A HOME REMEDY FOR PERSPIRING HANDS

Alum Cooler
Dissolve 2-1/2 tablespoons powdered alum in 1 pint hot

water. Cool the mixture. Apply it to the hands whenever needed, letting it dry on them.

QUICK HAND SOFTENERS

A hand softener need not be complicated. Certain basic ingredients can be pulled out of the cupboard or refrigerator and used almost as is to make hands soft and supple. Olive oil is a good emollient, as is cocoa butter or a combination of equal parts lanolin and petroleum jelly liberally rubbed into the hands after they have been immersed in water. Soaking hands in a bowl of fresh milk, buttermilk, or water and oatmeal or bran also helps them when they are rough and red. Surprisingly simple is this trick to soften hands: Merely push them down into a box of rough oatmeal (uncooked, of course). Oatmeal is really a wonder food for beauty, softening and giving a healthy glow to all parts of the body.

Palavi Patal's Potato Softener
This recipe, Palavi tells me, has been a tradition with the women of India for many years. Palavi's hands are beautiful, a testimony to the usefulness of the standard potato to soften hands. Cut a potato in half and rub it over your hands whenever you think about it, but particularly after they've been immersed in water. The potato removes kitchen odors from the hands too.

Gertrude's Grapefruit Softener
My downstairs neighbor Gertrude uses grapefruit peelings (the inside of them) to soften her hands. She scoops out the inside of a leftover breakfast grapefruit. Then after washing her hands or the dishes, she rubs the inside skin of the grapefruit over her hands, letting the natural oils seep into them.

HAND LOTIONS

Most of the following recipes originated in the last century, before commercial products were available. They serve to soften and ease rough, red hands, and they even combat wrinkles. Some will lighten freckles and other dark spots on the hands, as does Cornmeal Bleaching Paste (page 100).

Rose Water and Glycerin Lotion
Mix 1/2 teaspoon borax into 1 cup rose water (see page 154) until it dissolves. Add this mixture to 1 cup glycerin, stirring constantly. This lotion smooths and softens hands.

Honey and Lemon Juice Lotion
Carefully blend 1/4 cup each lemon juice, cologne, and honey. Put the mixture in a small bottle, shake well, and refrigerate. Use it to make the hands soft and fragrant.

Scented Almond Paste for the Hands

Pulverize enough almonds (whole or pieces) to make 1/2 pint almond meal. (I use a blender for this.) Beat 1 pint honey with 1 tablespoon egg yolk (about one egg yolk). Add to this mixture, little by little, 1 pint almond oil, then the almond meal, then 1-1/2 teaspoons essence of bergamot and then 1/2 teaspoon infusion of cloves (see page 157). Bottle the mixture, shake it well, and refrigerate it. Apply it to the hands to make them soft and scented.

Oatmeal Lotion

Mix together 1 teaspoon each olive oil, rose water (see page 154), cologne, and glycerin. Stir them into 1 quart warm water. Then slowly add 1/2 pound oatmeal, stirring all the while. Bottle and refrigerate the lotion. Rub it into the hands 3 times a day when they are acutely rough and red.

Lemon and Glycerin Lotion

Blend together 2 tablespoons glycerin and 2 tablespoons lemon juice. Put it into a small bottle, shake well, and refrigerate. Use the mixture to soften the hands and make them fragrant. Lemon traditionally is used to remove stains and the odors of garlic, onions, and other smelly foods. It's also a bleaching agent for freckles.

Orange Flower Water and Glycerin Lotion

Mix 1/2 teaspoon borax into 1 cup orange flower water until it dissolves. Then add the mixture to 1 cup glycerin, stirring constantly. Bottle this, shaking it well. Use it to soften hands.

THE GLOVE TREATMENT

In the last century and early in this one women were as likely to wear gloves filled with lotions to bed as they were to take hot water bottles to bed. These days, when wearing nightgowns is considered archaic, wearing gloves between the sheets may appear downright silly. But if your hands are seriously damaged—if you've ravaged them with paint remover or something equally deadly —you might choose to appear foolish for a night and rub your hands with one of the following concoctions to restore them to health. Then slip a pair of cotton gloves onto your hands and slide into bed—hopefully for one night unnoticed.

Gloved Barley Glop
Mix together 1/4 cup honey, 2 tablespoons glycerin, 1 cup barley flour, and 2 egg whites. Smear this on the hands and pull on a pair of gloves. Spend the night in them.

Gloved Almond Oil Glop
Beat 1/2 teaspoon egg yolk with 2 tablespoons almond oil and add 2 tablespoons rose water (see page 154). Smear this on the hands, and pull on a pair of gloves and sleep in them.

HAND MASSAGE

As are other parts of the body, the hands are massaged to release tension caused by overwork: typing, housework, anything that would task the hands. Massage relieves nervous tension and the ache caused by exposure to cold weather. When lotions and oils, even something as simple as olive oil, are massaged into the skin, they moisten and alleviate the dryness to which hands are so susceptible because of their constant exposure to water, detergents, and harsh weather.

Mme. Lina Cavalieri, a famous prima donna who

published a book called *My Secrets of Beauty* in 1914, in which she modestly by-lined herself as "the most famous living beauty," wrote this advice for hand massage. Assuming she was correct in her own assessment of her beauty, it may be wise to follow her treatment.

Mme. Cavalieri's Massage

"Fancy that you are wearing a pair of gloves for the first time. That you have accurately fitted the fingers and that you have now only to see that the gloves fit smoothly upon the back of the hands. You stroke the back of the right hand gently but firmly with the fingers of the left, and the left hand with the fingers of the right. Do this at least twenty times for each hand. Then lightly pinch the ends of each finger, pressing the sides of the fingers between the thumb and second finger."

When finger joints are sore, do the following: Pull at each of the fingers. Then with the thumb of the right hand on top of the left hand and two fingers beneath it, move from the wrist toward the fingers, massaging between the bones of the hand. Next, massage the finger joints one at a time. Do this several times. Repeat this for the right hand.

Another measure to take for stiff fingers is this: Spread them far apart and press them tightly down against a hard, flat surface. Press and release them several times.

HAND EXERCISES

Like massage, exercise relaxes your hands when they are stiff and tired from tension, overwork, or hazardous weather. Exercise also strengthens the hands so that they are less likely to become stiff and tired. And daily exercise could help to keep hands from developing a rheumatoid condition. Anything that stretches and flexes the fingers and tendons of the hands helps them. Many hand exercises can be improvised. These are a few that will start you on your way:

Hold the hands up at shoulder level. Let them drop at the wrists. Flap them back and forth swiftly from the wrists.

Pick up a rubber ball that fits your hand. Squeeze it tightly, then tighter. Put it down and pick it up again, repeating the process.

Play a make-believe piano, moving fast over the keyboard to flex the fingers. Stretch the fingers to reach an octave.

Stretch the hands open as wide as possible. Let them go limp and stretch them again.

Move the fingers across a table as if they were walking one after the other. Stretch them apart to take as big a "step" as possible.

NAILS

At six I quit biting my nails because I was promised two rabbits and a rabbit hutch. Next I quit biting my nails as an airline stewardess because I had to apply three coats of polish to my nails daily as part of training school regulations, and it seemed a shame to bite off all that work. Aside from that, the red polish signaled to me not to bite. I've outgrown rabbits and hutches, and I don't like red or any nail polish anymore, so the only way not to bite my nails, having a predilection to do so, is to get them as tough as shoe leather. The only way I know of to do this is to drink powdered gelatin in a glass of water—miserable to swallow but great insurance for strong nails.

Helena Rubinstein's Brittle Nail Formula

Helena Rubinstein said, back in 1930, that brittle nails could sometimes be helped if you dip them in a mixture of myrrh, lanolin, sweet almond oil, and white wax, all melted, as hot as you can stand it.

Mme. Rubinstein also suggested (being a practical lady) that to keep nails clean while doing grimy work one should scratch a bar of soap so that it edges under the nails, preventing any dirt from entering.

During Victorian times very elaborate and messy measures were taken to grow fingernails. Basically, with all these recipes the idea was to keep the nails lubricated. When dried from too much soaking in a dishpan or from the weather or from what-have-you, they become brittle and break. Here is a nineteenth century mutton lotion to build strong nails. Mutton is lanolin, remember?

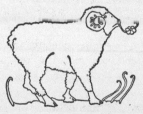

Mutton Lotion and Hog's Lard Pomade

Anoint nails with melted mutton fat that has been

mixed with the following pomade: Mix 1 teaspoon tar with 2 tablespoons hog's lard or melted pork fat. Rub the hands and nails with it, put on gloves, and wear them overnight. I'll stick to gelatin, thank you.

ROUGED NAILS

Before the cosmetics companies made a major business out of selling nail lacquer, women made their own. The color didn't blare out at you. It was soft and very feminine, usually buffed to a glow with cotton or a piece of chamois.

Nineteenth Century Nail Rouge

Carefully blend 1/2 teaspoon finely powdered carmine into 1 teaspoon fresh lard. Follow with 12 drops oil of bergamot. Rub this into the nails with cotton to give a soft, rosy tint. Obtain carmine at an artist's supply store selling unmixed pigments. Or buy cochineal which is the same as carmine, at an old-fashioned pharmacy (see Appendix).

A SEVENTEENTH CENTURY
RECIPE FOR HAND LOTION

This charming old recipe contains many of the same natural ingredients we still use today, proving this: Once you have a good thing, stick with it.

Paste for ye Hands

"Take a pound of sun raysens, stone and take a pound of bitter Almonds, blanch ym and beat ym in a stone morter with a glass of sack take ye peel of one lemond, boyle it tender; take a qyart of milk, and a pint of Ale and make therewith a Posett [a hot drink made of milk curdled with ale or wine and usually spiced]; take all ye Curd and putt it to ye Almonds; yn putt in ye Rayson: Beat all these till they come to a fine paste, and put in a pott, and keep it for ye use."

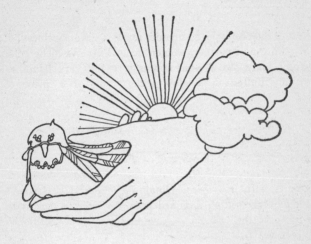

Footnotes:
Marigold,
Mint,
and
Lola Montez

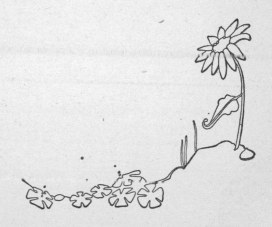

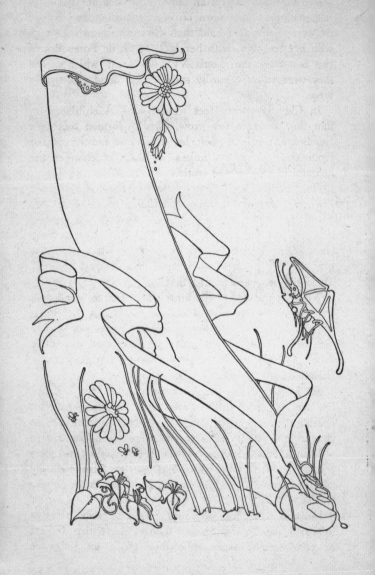

Mme. Vestris, a Victorian lady known for her beautiful feet, had her boots sewn on every morning and ripped off every night. It's said that she made more conquests with her feet than with her face. Mme. de Pompadour's two feet fitted into Louis XV's one hand, which means they were either absurdly small or his hand grotesquely large.

In China women's feet were bound at childhood so that they would never grow. This performed the same function as a chastity belt, for the women never ventured from their chambers unless carried. So changes the anatomical view of the erotic.

On the other hand that celebrated liberated lady Lola Montez—mistress to Bavaria's King Ludwig, friend to Franz Liszt and Alexandre Dumas, a woman who panned for gold, horsewhipped her enemies, and kept a bear on a chain—wrote in her book, *The Arts of Beauty*, published in 1853, "Better a bad bonnet than a shoe." There's a lot of sense to that.

Whereas the erotic qualities attributed to small feet were once entirely out of control, nowadays the liking for sturdy ones has gone to opposite extremes. Today men prefer their women with solid feet laced into army boots to carry them along the country's highways uncomplainingly.

To Leonardo da Vinci, the foot was "the greatest engineering device in the world." Yet feet take a sounder beating than any other part of the body. Evolution has not caught up with them. Not only were we not meant to walk upright on those twenty-six fragile bones (and some joints, ligaments, and muscles), but we also *certainly* were not meant to walk on the harsh concrete of city streets.

Imagine those feet of yours, meant to walk barefoot in earth, sand, and grass, taking the entire impact of your weight every time they touch an inflexible metropolitan sidewalk. Multiply that impact by all the steps taken each day, and look what an ordeal your feet have gone through. To contribute to the outrage done to our feet by civilized life, there are those monstrous fashions footwear manufacturers have contrived to keep themselves in business—although lately, I must admit, a few people, most of them health experts, have begun to design shoes that mold to the feet.

Feet, as Mme. Vestris discovered, deserve as much attention as your face. Treat them kindly, with massage, baths, and exercise. They work terribly hard.

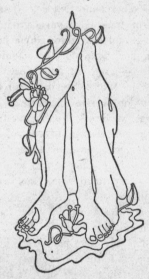

MASSAGE

Massaging and manipulating feet gets rid of aches, pains, and stiffness. Begin by rubbing the base of each toe with the ball of your thumb, in front and at the back, where they join the fat, cushiony part of your foot. Then pull each toe one at a time, little-piggy style. Rotate it around and around. Then massage each toe joint. Press your knuckled-up fist into the bottom of each foot, moving it in a circular motion. Give particular attention to the arches. Grab each foot one at a time with both hands, the fingers close together, pressing into and massaging the arch, the thumbs on the top of the foot, massaging downward from ankle to toes.

MASSAGE OILS AND OINTMENTS

Mint Ointment

Carefully mix 1/2 teaspoon peppermint extract with 1 teaspoon glycerin. Massage feet with this liquid for a cooling effect.

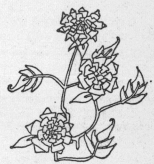

Marigold Massage Ointment

Early one spring my friend Sheila Weller, a lady who writes for *Rolling Stone*, brought me a pot of marigolds for my windowsill. When they had run their course, Sheila advised me to salvage the flowers and leaves and make a tea from them, rather than throw them out. The tea (with the flowers strained out) is mixed with yogurt or vegetable oil to make a massage cream for your feet. Traditionally marigolds were used to heal sprains, wounds, and varicose veins. Personally, I haven't seen them work in these three areas, but I know this ointment eases the aches in my feet. Marigolds also contain a coloring agent, calendula, which like carotene is a source of the skin food vitamin A.

Table Salt Massage Mixture

Put 1 cup table salt in an empty bathtub. Wet it slightly. Sit on the tub's edge and work the soles of the feet into the salt until they begin to soften up. Massage the salt into the heels, tops and sides of feet, and ankles wherever there is roughness. Rinse the feet off with cool water and dry them. This softens up calluses.

FOOT BATHS

Hot and Cold Foot Bath

Put the feet in the bathtub under the tap. Turn on the hot water and keep the feet under it as long as it's bearable. Then turn on the cold spigot and thrust the feet under that or rub ice over them. This takes courage, but the effect is ever so kind to tired, swollen feet.

Baking Soda Foot Bath

Soak feet in lukewarm water to which 1 tablespoon baking soda has been added. Much of the dead skin can be rubbed off with a towel. A pumice stone may be required to get the rest off.

Saltwater Foot Bath

Soak tired, swollen feet in warm saltwater, about 1 cup salt to 6 inches bathwater.

English Rosemary Foot Bath

A nineteenth century formula: Add 1 tablespoon rosemary to 1 gallon boiling water. Steep this, then strain off the liquid and cool it. The feet are immersed in the mixture for about 20 minutes. Warm water is added now and then as the water in the tub cools.

Juniper-Rosemary Foot Bath

Add 1 tablespoon each of rosemary, juniper berries, and mint to 1 gallon boiling water. Steep this to make a tea.

Strain off the liquid and cool it. Rosemary was once kept in oil, which was then used as a liniment to ease the pain of gout and rheumatism. Juniper berries were put on the burning coals that were used to heat schoolrooms in order to sweeten the air. This was a regular nineteenth century practice (this recipe dates from that time). Later it was found that the berries not only relieved the close atmosphere of those airtight old schools but also had a definite germicidal effect.

THREE MISCELLANEOUS FOOT SOOTHERS

Lemon Corn Plaster
Bind a slice of lemon to a corn overnight. Do this for several nights, and it's said that the corn will disappear.

Rice Foot Powder
Carefully mix 2 tablespoons powdered orris root, 6 tablespoons rice powder, and 1 tablespoon powdered alum. Keep this in an airtight container in a dry place. Apply it to feet to cool them.

Henna Foot Cooler
In India people powder their feet with henna in the summer to cool them.

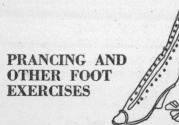

PRANCING AND OTHER FOOT EXERCISES

To strengthen arches and make feet flexible and relaxed when they're stiff, tired, or aching, grip a rolling pin or similar object with your feet, curving your toes around it. Or pick up pencils off the floor with your toes. Or stand, raise yourself to your toes, and prance like a pony.

To loosen stiff ankles move your feet around and around and up and down. Or move the left foot up and down so it says, "Yes, yes," simultaneously moving the right one from left to right so it says, "No, no." Then switch the feet, the left one saying, "No, no," while the right one says, "Yes, yes." It's rather like rubbing your tummy and patting your head at the same time. This is also a good exercise to test coordination.

To relax and strengthen your feet, knees, and legs pull your knees up, bringing the soles of your feet together. Grasp your hands around the outside of your feet and toes. Pull the toes up toward you. At the same time push your knees down toward the floor. This is great for knee joints and feet that have taken a beating on city pavements.

FOOTNOTE

Get your feet up whenever propriety permits. I used to sneak them up on the old chair opposite me in the library until a guard found me out. At home I often lie flat on the floor, a book in my hand and my feet up on the bed to drain fatigue out of the poor tortured things.

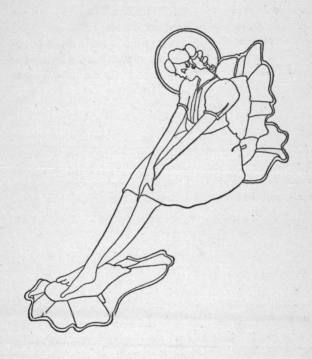

Eyes:
Elder Flowers,
Goldenseal Tea,
and
the Cherokees

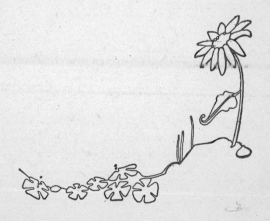

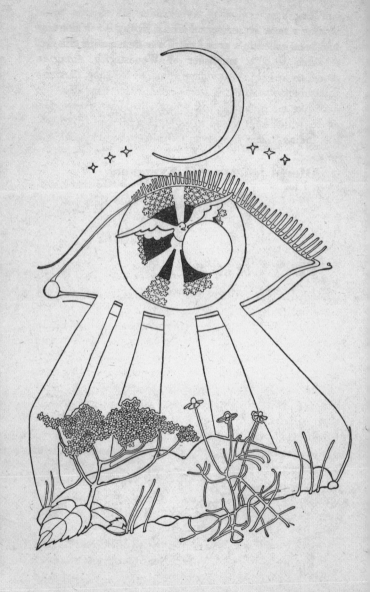

Not long ago, following an arduous six months spent writing a book on communal living, my eyes felt like they had been rolled in a gravel pit. I was bemoaning this fact to Allen Gordon, publisher of Woodstock's *Aquarian Angel*, as we sat in that village's famous tea shop, Norma's Squashblossom. Allen, it seems, shared the same affliction, since like me he had been turning out pages of type. His solace, which he credited to an eighteenth century Cherokee Indian remedy, was an infusion of goldenseal tea.

Allen's Goldenseal Eyewash

Steep 1 teaspoonful goldenseal tea in 1 pint boiling water. Cool the brew and filter it through cheesecloth. (All herbal eyewashes must have the residue strained off so it won't get into the eyes and irritate them.)

At about the same time, *The Rock Encyclopedia's* author, Lillian Roxon, recommended that I switch the color of my typing paper to alleviate my eyestrain. She reminded me that Colette wrote on blue paper, a fact I knew but thought to be a romantic conceit.

Another Woodstock friend, a practitioner of homeopathic medicine, verified the notion that white paper contributes to eyestrain, so I now write on pale blue, pink, or green paper. He also recommended vitamin A tablets to combat the eyestrain. Goldenseal tea, pastel paper, and vitamin A—aside from some eye exercises and sleep, which one Victorian said was the "best recipe for bright eyes"—are now my remedies.

Not everyone sits at the typewriter. But these days, with pollution outdoors, the glaring fluorescent lights indoors, the constant blinking of television, the bombardment of neon lights and other outgrowths of the technological age, it's a wonder our eyes don't take more of a beating than they do.

In the gentler days of gas and candlelight certain herbs and teas were used as eyewashes and poultices. They are being rediscovered today. Some I've used, some not, but for no other reason than that it's as impossible to get all of them as it would be to cook up all the food recipes one collects through the years.

All the preparations in this chapter have been tried by me or other people I know. But your eyes are *your* eyes. They react in their own specific manner. No eye remedy, I caution you, should be undertaken without your physician's recommendation.

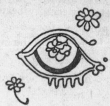

EYEWASHES

These serve to cleanse, tone, and strengthen the eyelids and internal parts of sore, red, irritated eyes.

Salt Eyewash
Dissolve a pinch of salt in 1/2 pint tepid water. Using an eyecup, bathe the eyes for a few minutes.

Mint Tea Eyewash
Brew some mint tea and dilute it with water. Use an eyecup to give the eyes a soothing menthol bath.

Elder Flower Eyewash

Claire Loewenfeld and Phillipa Back's wonderful book *Herbs, Health & Cookery* says that "elder flower water, an infusion, is safely used for eye and skin lotions."

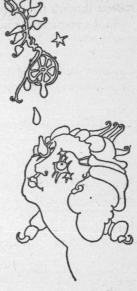

Rose Water Eyewash

A nineteenth century beauty book promises refreshing results from bathing the eyes in rose water (see page 154).

Orange Ouch Eye Bath

This one I wouldn't touch, simply because I've been treated to a squirt in the eye from my morning grapefruit. But Spanish ladies of last century calmly squeezed orange juice into their eyes to make them more brilliant.

EYE POULTICES

Eye poultices are usually some kind of medicated preparation applied to the exterior part of the eyes, either directly on the skin or via an antiseptic cloth or cotton pad to soothe them when they're aching, itching, sore, red, or tired.

Potato Poultice

A grated potato spread around the outside of the eyes and over the lids soaks into, soothes, and smooths tired delicate tissues while you nap.

125

Tea Bag Poultice
Apply a wet tea bag to each eye for 10 to 20 minutes while resting to reduce puffiness and circles.

Chamomile Tea Poultice
Make a tea of 1 part chamomile to 3 of hot water. Soak a cotton pad in this and put it on the eyes to reduce inflammation.

Ice Poultice
Rub ice cubes around the eyes to reduce their puffiness.

EYE CREAMS AND OILS

Generally, crow's-feet are caused by stress, eyestrain, strong sunlight, and squinting, the latter a great fault of nearsighted girls who refuse to wear glasses. Commercial eye creams are among the most expensive cosmetics, perhaps because they play upon the greatest of feminine fears, aging. The natural remedies listed below are effective and inexpensive. Basically, they work because they keep the tender, thin-skinned area around the eyes lubricated. Wrinkles are more likely to become implanted in dry skins.

Vitamin E Eye Oil
Vitamin E, all by itself, is an effective eye oil.

Carrot Eye Oil
Pulverize a carrot in the blender and add to it enough safflower oil to allow the grated vegetable to hold to the area around the eyes. This is helpful as a retarder of crow's-feet, as are cocoa butter and pure lanolin.

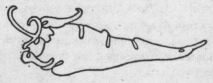

AN EYELASH GROWER, AN EYEBROW TONIC, AND AN EYEBROW DYE

Castor Oil Eyelash Grower
Applied each night to eyelashes, it helps them to grow.
Olive Oil Eyebrow Tonic
Like castor oil, olive oil will pick up the growth of scanty eyebrows.
Sage Tea Eyebrow Dye
Strongly brewed sage tea brushed onto the eyebrows is said to dye them.

EYE EXERCISES

To relieve eyestrain, move your eyes up, down, right, and left in a circular motion. Close them. Repeat the rolling process in the opposite direction. Another version of this is to move the eyes around the four corners of a wall.

To exercise the upper lids raise your eyebrows. While they are in that position, raise and lower your eyelids.

To focus the eyes fix them on a faraway object, then on a closer one. Look outward; move inward. Repeat the motion.

To firm up the eyelids open your eyes in a wide stare, then squeeze them tightly shut. Repeat this action several times.

To relax the eyes rub your hands together to create heat by friction. Place the palms against your eyes without applying pressure to the eyeballs. A warm, pleasant relaxation will seep through your eyes. This is an old yoga trick.

Teeth:
Table Salt,
Caraway Seeds,
and
Queen Victoria

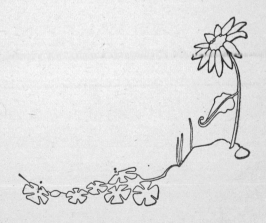

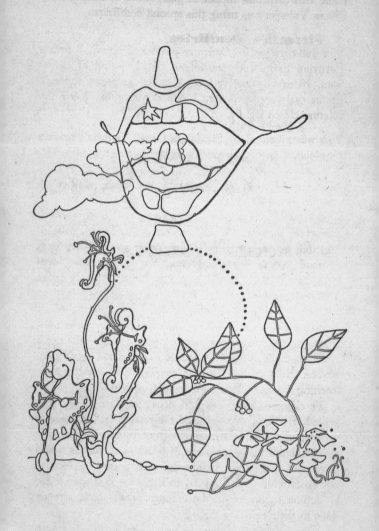

In Victorian times the Masai women of East Africa, renowned for the extreme beauty of their teeth, polished them with corncobs dipped in palm wine. Simultaneously Queen Victoria was using this special dentifrice:

Victoria's Dentifrice

Mix well together 1-1/2 drams powder of myrrh, 3 drams Peruvian bark, finely powdered, 10 drops oil of cinnamon, 10 drops oil of cloves, 1 ounce prepared chalk, 2 drams orris root powder, 1 ounce rose pink. Keep the mixture closed tightly.

This was prepared by Sir James Clark, Victoria's private physician. (And it's probably better to leave it with Victoria. Other usable recipes follow.) George Washington, on the other hand, must have done something wrong: He wore false teeth.

Marlene Dietrich said that all a woman really needs are good legs and a full set of teeth. And Voltaire said that no woman can be bad looking with good teeth or good looking with bad ones. My dentist, who loves teeth, agrees with Marlene and Voltaire. Nobody looks pretty with bad teeth.

I once accused my dentist of having a painting of an extracted molar on his office wall. He said that was nonsense; it was an abstract something or other. I still think it's a tooth. Anyway, he knows more about teeth than anyone. He should write this chapter, but he's too busy teaching his patients about preventive dentistry.

It's claimed tooth loss and decay can be totally prevented if people will care for their teeth in the manner prescribed by the American Dental Association. My dentist could put himself out of business if people would listen and teach their children proper dental habits, but not everyone listens. Besides, he'll have enough work for a lifetime fixing up all the damage people have already done to their teeth.

HOW TO SAVE YOUR TEETH AND CUT DOWN ON DENTAL BILLS TOO

Preventive dentistry basically teaches proper home dental care. The premise of this book is that practically everything from making face creams to cutting hair can be done at home. It would be folly to suggest you'll never have to see your dentist again if you follow these measures—you *must* see him if only to verify that you've done a good job—but preventive dentistry, combined with dental checkups, can save you an amazing number of dollars.

These are the facts: Early in 1972 the important contribution of plaque to tooth decay was discovered. Plaque is a colorless film that forms and always has formed on everyone's teeth, even Queen Victoria's. Plaque houses bacteria that produce tooth- and gum-destroying acids, toxins, and enzymes.

Food helps bacteria adhere to plaque colonies on the teeth. Bacteria need food to survive, and they particularly love sugar, which in the mouth becomes dextran, a stubbornly adhesive substance. Dextran hugs bacteria even tighter to your teeth so they can do their dirty work.

Plaque, with its colonies of bacteria, performs its most active damage in the first twenty minutes after eating. By brushing after meals and snacks, the bacteria-infested plaque is broken up, greatly reducing the chance of its eroding and decaying your teeth.

Sugar is deadly, but if you're absolutely addicted to it, eat sweets following meals so the sticky mass can conveniently be brushed off afterward. Research has found that people with the most cavities are snackers who brush only after meals.

CLEANING YOUR TEETH WITH STYLE

Brush within the first twenty minutes after eating, when mouth bacteria are doing their heaviest damage. Place the toothbrush, a soft one (a hard one won't get bacteria off any more efficiently, and it's likely to irritate gums), on its side at the top of your gums, inside your lips, bristles facing upward. Shimmy the bristles back and forth slowly, moving downward toward the tooth enamel, until they are standing straight on the actual tooth. Move the brush on down to the tip of the tooth. Repeat the same motion on the bottom teeth, but move the brush upward. Don't move the brush quickly back and forth, pushing the gums down like cuticles.

Dental floss sneaks out food particles caught between your teeth where the brush can't reach them. Snap a piece of floss out of the container. It should be long enough for you to wrap it around the index finger of each hand and still have a piece two to three inches long in the middle. Move the floss up and down (gently—don't saw) between each tooth and into the V-shaped gum area.

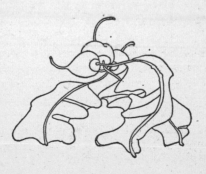

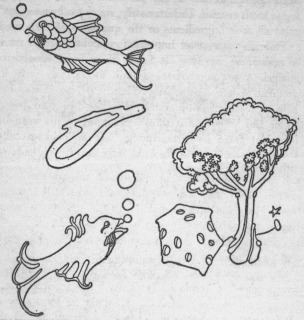

EAT WELL FOR GOOD TEETH

Vitamins and minerals—specifically vitamin D and calcium—combat tooth decay and build strong gums. The sun is vitamin D's best source, but it's also present in mackerel, salmon, herring, tuna, and sardines, and frequently milk is fortified with it. Yellow cheese, cottage cheese, milk, molasses, almonds, turnip greens, and broccoli provide calcium.

TABLE SALT, CINNAMON, AND OTHER TEETH CLEANERS

The market is filled with toothpastes, each promising to

outdo the others. Those that will have you smiling ultra-white contain abrasives and peroxide, which are damaging to tooth enamel. Unfortunately, many toothpastes don't print all their ingredients or the quantities of each used.

Fluoride is the most important contribution ever made to preventive dentistry. It fights plaque and strengthens enamel. A few toothpastes contain this as an active ingredient. Some cities—New York, for one—have fluoride in their drinking water. If it's not in your town's water and your dentist thinks you need it, it's available in tablet form by prescription. Not so coincidentally, toothpastes containing fluoride have a printed endorsement from the American Dental Association on the package.

Table Salt Tooth Cleaner

Table salt is my favorite dentifrice. I drink tea passionately and so end up with dingy brown teeth. But salt and my toothbrush make them white again. Salt also removes berry stains. And friends who smoke, taking my advice about salt, have rid themselves of ugly nicotine stains. Aside from its whitening quality, common salt has an antiseptic effect that is particularly repugnant to plaque. Salt is also a good deodorizer. And a little table salt can

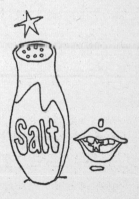

be packed off to the ladies' room after you eat a meal out if you want to be efficient about brushing your teeth. Some people mix equal quantities of baking soda and salt for a dentifrice. I prefer the taste of salt, but each to her own.

Etienne's Orange and Lemon Peel Paste

A friend I met years ago in Switzerland taught me to use pulverized (use a blender) dried lemon and orange peel in a regular dentifrice to whiten the teeth and sweeten the breath. The peel can also be mixed with salt or baking soda.

Wintergreen Toothpaste

Mix 1 teaspoon of wintergreen and 1/2 cup baking soda with 1 cup water for a fragrant whitening toothpaste.

Peppermint Toothpaste

Blend 1/4 cup baking soda with 2 drops oil of peppermint for a whitening menthol toothpaste.

Cinnamon Toothpaste

Blend 2 tablespoons baking soda and 2 tablespoons cinnamon with 2 tablespoons oil of cinnamon for a tangy cleaner.

KISS, KISS: BREATH FRESHENERS

Table salt or baking soda mixed in a glass of water, as strong as you can take it, is the mouthwash I find most effective and inexpensive. Gargling with table salt mouthwash is soothing for a sore throat too. Chewing parsley sprigs sweetens breath, as does chewing watercress, which like parsley is loaded with natural chlorophyll. The water from boiled watercress, cooled and swished around in the mouth, is a very old American remedy to cure bleeding gums. Orange flower tea makes a pleasant and effective mouthwash, as do rose water (see page 154) and clove tea mouthwash, first used around the time of the Civil War.

Clove Tea Mouthwash

Infuse 3 tablespoons cloves (bruised or sliced) and 1 pint boiling water in a covered vessel for 1 hour. When it's cold, filter off the liquid to make an excellent deodorizing mouthwash.

Brandy-Spearmint Mouthwash

Mix together 1/2 cup brandy, 1/2 cup spearmint tea, and 1 teaspoon salt for a fragrant, tangy mouthwash. This must have been a favorite of Victorian gentlemen, since it gave them a chance to tipple on the side with legitimate reason.

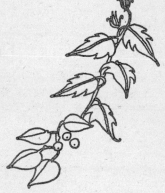

MASTICATORIES

Masticatories are old cleaning devices that more often than not produced some euphoric side effects. Arnold Cooley, in a mid-nineteenth century beauty book, records that masticatories were "employed as intoxicants, medicinals, and cosmetics, most of them with the first intention. In Europe, it was generally tobacco, in Turkey and

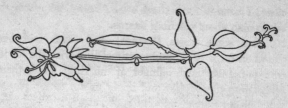

several Eastern nations Opium. In Indian and neighboring Asiatic nations betel or betel nuts, whilst in some other part of the world preparations of cacao are employed. As cosmetics Orris root, Cinnamon and Sandalwood are frequently chewed to scent the breath."

Snackers are advised by the American Dental Association to switch from soft candy, which creeps into tooth crevices, to carrots, raw broccoli, celery, nuts, and seeds, masticatory foods with natural cleaning actions. Try chewing Korean ginseng root, also said to be an aphrodisiac, an added bonus.

People in the past seem to have been as obsessed by clean breath as we are today, although they didn't have television to remind them of it. Liquor, of course, has always been a major breath offender. Husbands were as eager to cover up telltale booze breath then as they are now. Gin shops in the mid-nineteenth century graciously provided a supply of caraway seeds and lemon peel to imbibers—not only husbands but also wives, daughters, servants, and working people who patronized them. I've used both the caraway seeds and the lemon peel. They taste good and do the job.

TO EXTRACT A TOOTH PAINLESSLY

Here's a folk remedy that once worked for a far-gone hobgoblin, quoted in Maurice Richards' *Brews and Po-*

tions. I wouldn't try it on a bet, being, of course, very squeamish about catching lizards.

"Find some newts [lizards] and some foul beetles found on ferns in the summertime. Pulverize the lot in an iron pot. Lick the forefinger of the right hand, then insert it into the powder and apply to the tooth. The tooth will fall out immediately without pain."

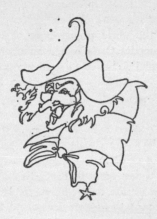

Fragrances:
Potpourri,
Lemon Extract,
and
the Queen of Hungary

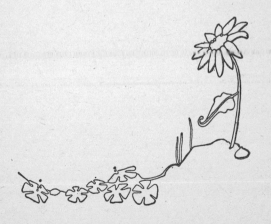

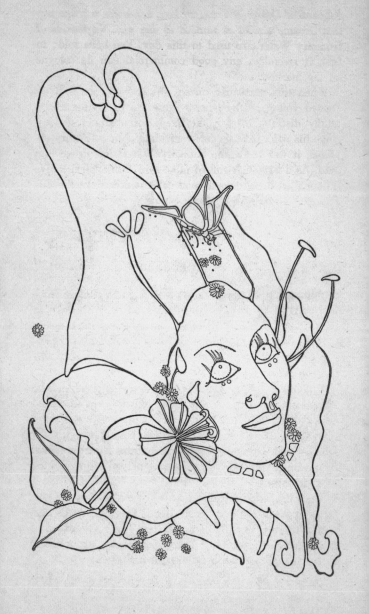

A beautiful Queen of Hungary long ago made a fragrance that became almost as famous as she was. Variations of Hungary Water are used to this day, I've been told; in fact, it resembles any good commercial eau de cologne on the market now.

When this particular queen was seventy, she still attracted young lovers. One, a mere lad of eighteen, was totally distraught when the aged queen would not become his wife. It all sounds very kinky, but as history explains, it was really the Hungary Water that drove him mad. As a British friend of mine said with typical native humor, "In those days a good cologne did make the difference."

Hungary Water

This recipe is really too expensive and troublesome to make. It calls for 1/2 ounce oil of rosemary, 2 drams oil of lavender, 30 grains oil of petit grain, 3 drams tincture of tolu, 1/2 pint orange flower water, and 5 ounces rectified spirits. No specific instructions on what to do with these ingredients are available. But if you want to go to all the bother, note that the recipe serves a dual purpose. As Hungary Water passed through history, ladies of distinction began to tipple it.

Perfumed, incensed, and odoriferous ointments have existed since antiquity. The Bible tells of the Wise Men who brought gifts of frankincense and myrrh to the infant Jesus. The Egyptians anointed their slave girls for months before they were sold into harems, as it increased their value. And Roman orgies were played out in a thick mist of incense.

The Elizabethan era brought in a new passion for perfume. It was certainly Elizabeth the Virgin Queen's passion. She wore a string of pomanders (balls composed of ambergris, benzoin, and other perfumes) around her neck and another frequently about her girth.

Perfumed leathers were brought to England in 1550, when the Earl of Oxford returned from Italy with scented gloves for his queen. Each glove was trimmed with four roses of colored silk. Elizabeth was so pleased that she wore them when she had her portrait painted and called them the Earl of Oxford's perfume.

The queen's own perfume recipe is still in existence, should you be able to find the ingredients and want to keep royal company.

The Virgin Queen's Perfume

The recipe calls for: "8 grains Musk, put into 8 spoonfuls Rosewater with 3 spoonfuls of Damask Water and a quarter of an oz. of sugar. Boil 5 hours and strain."

Musk, as well as ambergris, favorite animal essences, are now available only in synthetic form, as the price for the real thing is prohibitive. Musk grain from the Himalayan musk deer costs three thousand dollars per pound. It is difficult to discern what Damask Water might have been. One chemist suggests it was pure water from a particular district called Damask, something like distilled water. Again, it may have been the liquid from Damask roses, but then the total quantity of rose water should be 11 spoonfuls. Even so, this should make a nice fragrance, although not exactly like the queen's.

Doubtless strong essences were necessary in those days before baths were convenient; they were so important, in fact, that special places called still rooms, where fragrances were prepared, became a part of every castle and estate. Gloves were impregnated with perfumes, as were handkerchiefs, shoes, hemlines, wigs, and bedclothes. Perfumed necklaces and rings were worn.

Napoleon's Empress Joséphine wore a musk perfume so strong it permeated her bedroom walls. It is reported that tourists who pass through the room can still smell it.

Strong, heady fragrances belong to another time. Now

that the middle class has moved into tepees, with copies of *The Whole Earth Catalog* for pillows, scents have been created to suit a natural way of life. Now people want to smell like all outdoors—like herbs, fruits, flowers, and woods.

My friend Mary Orser, who has her M.A. in psychology and her heart in astrology, wears the scent of wild honey. Phaedre, who lives with Ytar and baby Noa in Mary's house, wears a cologne made of vodka and cinnamon bark. And I have grown accustomed to Ehler's lemon extract, about thirty-five cents at the supermarket.

Other food extracts make surprisingly nice fragrances. I know people who happily use peppermint, vanilla, or almond extract. Food extracts have one shortcoming: They are slight on staying power so may have to be reapplied more frequently than costlier scents. Some supermarket scents are:

Pure almond extract (30% alcohol)
Pure anise extract (70% alcohol)
Pure orange extract (80% alcohol)
Pure lemon extract (80% alcohol)
Pure peppermint extract (70% alcohol)
Pure vanilla extract (35% alcohol)

More sophisticated natural scents in essential oil form are available at health food stores, herbalists, apothecaries, and head shops (see Appendix).

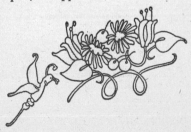

In considering what essential oils to buy, it is important to know the quantities in which they are sold. Many old-fashioned recipes, although quaint to read, may prove expensive to make if the oils cannot be bought in small enough quantities. The firms listed in the Appendix have mail-order catalogs in which availabilty and price can be checked out ahead of preparation.

Unfortunately, fragrance ingredients are generally more expensive than the staple items frequently used for recipes in other chapters, but then fragrances have always been considered a luxury. And you may hit upon the most exotic scent yet to be discovered once you begin experimenting.

Some of the fragrant oils listed in the catalogs are:

Basil
Bay leaf
Bergamot (from the fresh rind of the bergamot orange, grown in southern Europe)
Caraway
Cardamom
Carnation
Celery seed
Cinnamon
Clove
Eucalyptus
Freesia
Honeysuckle
Jasmine
Lavender
Lime
Narcissus
Neroli (Orange blossom)
Nutmeg

Peppermint
Petit grains
Rose geranium
Rosemary
Sandalwood (from the fragrant wood of an evergreen tree grown in southern India or one found in Hawaii, called yellow or citron sandalwood)
Spearmint
Sweet pea
Tuberose
Verbena (from leaves that give off a lemony scent)
Violet
Ylang ylang (from flowers of a Malayan tree)
(I have been told that certain rare oils—tolu, for example—can be specially ordered.)

These oils can be used directly on the skin, diluted to

make a cologne or toilet water, or mixed to make some of the fragrance recipes in this chapter.

One delectable way to use them comes from Victorian times:

To Perfume Drawers

Rub the fragrance—sandalwood, rose geranium, eucalyptus, or any other of your choice—inside your bureau drawers to give a fragrant odor to your clothes. It's nice to match the scent to the one worn on your skin.

The fragrant oils can also be mixed in with a plain, inexpensive, mildly scented powder—Mennen's or Johnson's Baby—to make a sweet-smelling after-bath talc.

White Rose Powder

Mix together 1/2 teaspoon attar of roses (or tuberose) and 1 teaspoon oil of bergamot (or neroli). Gradually add them to 1 pound white unscented (or slightly scented) powder, rubbing it all together until it's thoroughly mixed.

Maceration, expression, and enfleurage (a French method used in the famous Grasse perfumeries) are the usual techniques for extracting oils from flowers, fruits, herbs, and barks.

MACERATION

Maceration can be achieved in two ways. One method is to rub the ingredient (a particularly strong one like eucalyptus or mint) between your hands and then over your body for the instant fragrant sensation. The scent may linger, depending upon the weather, the quality of your skin, and other elements. Whenever I rub eucalyptus between my palms, I have an instant memory of my California childhood, when those pulverized leaves first produced their quick magical odor. Lauren Hutton, the beautiful actress and model, has the same feeling for fresh garden mint. She crushes it, then smooths it on her hair.

A more sophisticated maceration process is one in which the scented flower or herb is soaked in oil or glycerin in an airtight container. Small well-washed jars and bottles work well for this purpose. The proportions of fragrance base are usually 1 part flower petals, herbs, or spices to 4 parts oil or glycerin.

The oil can be vegetable or mineral. Mineral—baby oil, for example—is good to use. Vegetable oils are also usable, but their odor (that of olive oil, in particular) may interfere with the fragrance you want. Vegetable oils also turn rancid if the fragrance mixture is not refrigerated. Or you may unwittingly use a spoiled vegetable oil, not knowing you have done so until the rancid scent has overtaken the one planned. I once ruined a batch of flower fragrance with a rancid safflower oil I took to be fresh. If you do use vegetable oil, safflower is best, as its scent is the most innocuous. But it should be bought fresh. I prefer to use glycerin for the maceration process.

It is generally true that the longer the fragrance ingredient sits in the oil or glycerin, the stronger the scent will become. A month is usually not too long. Sometimes if the fragrance is slow to take, it can sit even longer. But again, when it's a particularly strong fragrance, like rosemary or mint, I may use it the same day or the day after.

Heat helps the fragrance to permeate the oil or glycerin. Let the container sit in the sun for a while. Or place it in a basin or pan of hot water, renewing the water when it cools. This can take thirty minutes or longer. Cloves seem to follow the opposite rule: They should sit in a cool place.

Flowers should always be pulled off their stems before they are put in the oil. Herbs and spices seem to give a stronger odor when used in their original form: cinnamon bark, for example, or unbruised cloves. Pulverize the cinnamon yourself and bruise the cloves. Rub rosemary between your fingers to bring out its fragrance before tossing it in the bottle.

Once the lot is mixed together, it can be tossed in the blender to thoroughly integrate the fragrance ingredient with the oil. Shake the bottle daily to keep the residue from settling on the bottom and not permeating the oil. Flower or other materials may be strained out of the oil through a sieve or cheesecloth. Good materials for maceration are:

Herbs and Spices	Flowers	Tree Leaves and Needles
Rosemary	*Carnations*	*Eucalyptus*
Cinnamon	*Lavender*	*Pine*
Cloves	*Gardenias*	
Peppermint	*Roses*	
Cardamom		
Nutmeg		
Caraway seeds		

I have also heard that cassia, violets, acacia, mignonette, and orange flowers hold their fragrance. It's also a fact that yellow roses retain fragrance better than red ones unless the latter are hothouse-grown.

There are also two old-fashioned maceration methods that sound time-consuming, but since they take so long, they may produce stronger, more lasting fragrances.

Old-Fashioned Maceration No. 1

Oil (mineral, vegetable) or glycerin is put into a stainless steel or heatproof glass pan set in a pan of boiling salted water. Flowers are picked from their stems, torn apart, dropped into the oil, and allowed to macerate for 1 to 2 hours over low heat. The mixture is set aside for 24 hours, after which the flowers are taken out and drained. Fresh flowers take their place, and the process is repeated until the oil is fragrant.

Old-Fashioned Maceration No. 2

Oil is placed in a stainless steel or heatproof glass pan, warmed to about 130 degrees Fahrenheit by setting it in a shallow pan containing hot but not boiling water. The flowers to be extracted are enclosed in muslin bags, then placed in the oil or glycerin, where they stay for 1/2 to 2 days. The bags are taken out, drained, pressed, refilled with fresh flowers, and returned to the pan sitting in another container of hot water. This procedure is repeated 12 to 16 times or more to give a highly scented oil- or glycerin-based substance.

ENFLEURAGE

The process of enfleurage uses only the heat of the sun to extract the fragrance. Uniformly sized pieces of glass framed in wood (perhaps glassed picture frames) are used. Each piece of glass is covered with a thin layer of a greasy, unscented substance or glycerin, over which the flowers are strewn. The frames are piled on top of each other to exclude air and insects. The flowers are renewed every 24 hours until the glycerin is sufficiently impregnated with the fragrance. It is then scraped from the glass, melted by gentle heat, and strained. The fragrance is called French pomade. A cruder form of this method was used by the perfumers of India. The flowers were alternated with layers of sesamum, related to sesame seed, and kept airtight in a cloth. In this country poppy seeds were used this way.

EXPRESSION

Expression is used in obtaining citrus fruit oils, especially lemon and lime. I have also tried orange and grapefruit, and although the extracted oils are wonderful for the skin, they fail to have the pungent odor of lemon or lime—at least, I have no luck securing it. Professional perfumers may do better.

Oils are traditionally expressed from citrus rinds by a press. My citrus rinds are expressed by two methods: Grating them by hand or cutting the rinds into small pieces and running them through a blender. To the pulverized rind I add the fruit's juice and a few drops of glycerin or baby oil. I press the whole through a sieve, then return it to the blender, where it becomes a creamy skin fragrance and a good hand lotion. The pulverized pieces left in the sieve can be used on the face and hands to lubricate the skin and restore its acid mantle. This essence is best preserved in the refrigerator in an airtight bottle.

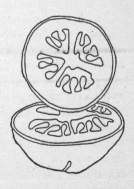

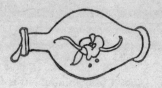

ALCOHOL

Securing the proper alcohol is a problem. It's best to use pure grain alcohol, which is 100%, or to use 95% or 90% alcohol, which is slightly diluted. It is illegal to sell these in many places, at least without a prescription. I live in New York and can't buy it even with a prescription, although it's sold in neighboring New Jersey and Connecticut without one. I can buy it in Vermont with a prescription, but am limited to a fifth at a time. But I have been told that some benevolent pharmacist might sell you the contraband alcohol if you can't get it elsewhere and if he knows you well. I have also been told not to mention this, for it's against the law. You can go blind drinking pure or nearly pure grain alcohol, and some people will drink anything, even their perfume.

Since pure grain alcohol is out unless I cross the border to Connecticut or am in Vermont, three other solutions are available to me, and to you if you're in the same situation: 1. Vodka, 40% alcohol, in most places. In some locales it is 50%. 2. Rubbing alcohol, 70%. 3. Perfume diluent. I know that this is distributed by Caswell-Massey (see Appendix for address), but send for other store catalogs (addresses listed in Appendix) to see if they sell diluents also. I suggest assembling catalogs and comparing prices before ordering.

Perfume diluent is probably the best of the three solutions to the problem, although the most expensive. However, I prefer vodka. Although its odor is strong at first, it evaporates. Rubbing alcohol evaporates in the air too, but its odor is stronger than vodka's.

I'm telling you about the various available alcohols now, since the recipes that follow simply call for "alcohol." The kind you use is your choice.

EXTRACTS

You can make extracts by pouring alcohol over the pomades and oils secured from the processes of maceration, enfleurage, and expression. The alcohol is added in varying proportions, depending upon the strength of the pomade.

Nineteenth Century Violet Extract
Pour 2 parts alcohol over 1 part violet pomade.

INFUSIONS

Infusion is a process for making a fragrance without using a fragrant oil-like base. It involves steeping a fragrance in a liquid but not boiling it. Think of the way tea is made, and you have the idea. The fragrance ingredient—cloves, rosemary, lavender flowers—can be steeped in alcohol, vinegar, or water.

With infusion as with maceration, it generally holds

true that the longer an ingredient sits in a liquid, the stronger the scent becomes. You can also help infused fragrances to take hold by putting them in the sun or warm water. There are some exceptions to this: Cloves, for example, should not sit in a liquid for longer than 5 to 6 days, and the mixture should be kept in a cool place.

AROMATICS

Essentially, aromatics are made with spices and herbs infused in vinegar, resulting in a heady, pungent odor. In the last century a woman's aromatic vinegar was as much an insignia as her perfume is today. The vinegar infusion had a twofold purpose for her: It served both as her fragrance and as a facial astringent known as cosmetic vinegar (see page 55).

FLOWER WATERS

Flower waters are made by simmering petals over a low flame in much the same way as you would cook spinach. Little water is used, the petals producing their own liquid. The method used in the following recipe will work with flowers other than roses.

Rose Water

You will need 3 pounds rose petals altogether. Place 2 to 3 cups petals in a glass or enamel saucepan. Add just enough water to prevent them from burning. Cover the pan and cook the petals over a very low flame, simmering the mixture for 30 to 40 minutes. Then remove the petals from the pan and replace them with an equal amount of fresh petals. Try not to add more water; there should be an increased amount of liquid from the first batch of petals. Keep repeating this process until all the petals have been used. Strain the liquid through cheesecloth into airtight glass jars. Store the jars for 3 days before using the contents. Each pound of petals should produce 1 pint rose water. Initially, you could try this recipe with a smaller quantity of rose petals—say 1 pound.

DISTILLATION

Distillation produces a strong-scented flower water. The following equipment is needed: an enamel teakettle with a spout and a tight lid, a piece of rubber tubing 4 feet long, a glass jar with an airtight lid, and a pan filled with cold water.

Fill the teakettle 1/2 full of water. Fit one end of the rubber tubing over the teakettle spout. The other end of the tubing goes into the jar. The middle section of tubing rests in the pan of cold water. Turn the heat on very low under the teakettle. Fill the kettle with flower petals, stirring them into the water. Then cover the kettle. When the petals have been reduced in bulk by simmering them, add more until you have used 1 pound of them. The tubing will fill up with steam from the spout, which will condense into liquid at the point where the tubing passes through the pan of cold water. Flower water will drip from the end of the tube into the glass jar. When the water has stopped dripping into the jar, cover it tightly. Keep the distillate 2 or 3 days before using. The distillation method produces a stronger fragrance than the process used to make flower water.

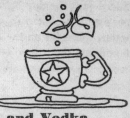

FRAGRANCE RECIPES

Phaedre's Cinnamon and Vodka Cologne

Pulverize enough cinnamon bark to fill an airtight container 1/6 full (or a little more). Fill the rest of the container (an empty spice jar will do) with 80% vodka. Shake it every day. It can be used immediately, but the longer it sits, the stronger the fragrance becomes. The pieces of bark may or may not be strained out, as you wish. Cinnamon has a lovely pungent odor. And it's said to have antiseptic qualities, the scent having the power to destroy many infectious microbes. When mixed with glycerin, cinnamon also makes a terrific scented bath oil or preparation.

Susie's California Cologne

Susie Olquin, one of those great-looking tall California blondes and a friend of mine, mastered this recipe in her kitchen at Manhattan Beach. Citrus peels are reduced to grated pieces or small sliced slivers in order to measure them.

> 2 cups fresh rose petals
> 2 cups alcohol
> 6 tablespoons fresh lemon peel
> 6 tablespoons fresh lime peel
> 6 tablespoons fresh orange peel
> 1/4 cup dried basil
> 1/4 cup dried rosemary
> 1/4 cup dried peppermint leaves

Soak the rose petals for 1 week in the alcohol in a tightly

lidded jar. The day before the week is up, put the citrus peels and the herbs in a pan and cover with the boiling water. Put a lid on the mixture. The next day strain the liquid into the rose solution (having first strained out the rose petals). Shake well.

OLD-FASHIONED FRAGRANCE RECIPES

Infusion of Cinnamon and Cloves
Combine 3 tablespoons broken-up cinnamon sticks, 1-1/2 tablespoons cloves, bruised, and 1 pint alcohol. Let this stand in a warm, dark place for 1 week. Shake it frequently during that time. Strain off the liquid in this recipe, and in all those following that use solid materials such as spices or flowers.

Infusion of Cloves
Mix 1 part cloves, crushed or powdered coarsely, with 5 parts alcohol. Allow this to stand at a low temperature for 5 to 6 days—longer than that and the liquid will become murky.

Infusion of Coriander
Infuse together for 1 month 2 parts well-crushed coriander seed and 9 parts alcohol.

Lavender Water No. 1
Combine 1 part lavender flower and 4 parts alcohol. Let the infusion stand for 1 month's time at most.

Lavender Water No. 2
Combine 2 tablespoons oil of lavender, 2 tablespoons oil of bergamot, 4 bruised cloves, 1 pint alcohol; shake well. Let this stand 1 month. Then add 1/4 cup distilled water and, if you wish, about 1/3 teaspoon essence of musk or ambergris, which increases the scent's longevity.

Eau de Marechale
Mix together 2 tablespoons oil of violet, 1-1/2 tablespoons

oil of cloves, and 1-1/2 tablespoons oil of bergamot. Add the mixture to 1 pint alcohol, and let this sit for 1 week. Then add 1/2 pint orange flower water. Shake the mixture well. Keep it in a tightly lidded jar.

Sir James Clark's Aromatic Vinegar
As was mentioned in the Chapter on teeth, Sir James Clark was Queen Victoria's private physician, so it's reasonable to assume she used this recipe.

Combine 2 tablespoons dried rosemary, 2 tablespoons dried sage, 2 tablespoons dried lavender flowers, 1 teaspoon bruised cloves, 1 teaspoon camphor, and 1-1/2 pints distilled vinegar. Keep the mixture in the hot sun for 2 weeks, or warm it several times over a low flame during the same period of time. Filter it before using.

Thyme Aromatic
Mix together 1 scant teaspoon oil of mint, 1 scant teaspoon oil of lavender, 1 scant teaspoon oil of rosemary, and 1 scant teaspoon oil of lemon. Add to them 3 tablespoons alcohol. Add the lot to an infusion of thyme (similar to the infusion of coriander: see page 157).

POTPOURRI

Potpourri is a mixture of dried flower petals, citrus rinds, and other such spices, which is kept in a covered jar for the fragrance that fills a room when the lid is lifted.

A Very Old Potpourri
Gather rose petals in the early morning. Toss them onto a table in a cool, airy place to lie until the dew has dried off, then put them in a large stone jar, sprinkling a little salt over 1/2-inch layers of petals. Add to your pile of petals from morning to morning until enough roses for your purpose have been gathered. Let them stand in the

jar for 10 days after the last are gathered, stirring the whole every morning. Have 2 tablespoons each cloves, coarsely ground allspice, and stick cinnamon that has been broken and shredded fine with the fingers. Transfer the petals to another jar and scatter the mixed-together spices in layers alternately with the petals. Cover the jar tightly and let it stand in a dark place for 3 weeks, when the stock will be ready for a permanent jar. Have ready 1/2 tablespoon each mace, allspice, and cloves, all coarsely ground, 1/2 dried nutmeg, 1 tablespoon cinnamon, broken fine, 2 tablespoons powdered orris root, and 1/4 pound dried lavender flowers. Mix all together in a bowl and proceed to fill the rose jar with alternate layers of stock and this last mixture. A few drops each of several essential oils—rose geranium, neroli, and bitter almond —should be sprinkled on the layers as you progress. Over the whole pour 2 tablespoons fine cologne or rose water (see page 154). This is sufficient to fill 2 1-quart jars or one very large jar, and it will keep for years. Occasionally various sweet things may be added—a few leaves of lemon, for example. If the jar is left open 1/2 hour each day, it will fill your room with a delicate, exquisite aroma.

Katora's Santa Cruz Potpourri

My friend Katora Leibheardt, a sixty-seven-year-old grandmother who lives in Santa Cruz, California, with 175 rose bushes, has a simple recipe for potpourri. She gathers her rose petals and puts them with orange peels and cloves in a large pan on top of her old wood-burning stove. The heat from the stove brings out the fragrance of the potpourri, and the kitchen is sweet with it. Katora gathers up small portions of the mixture and puts them into tiny matchboxes to give to friends and neighborhood children to smell. She gave a little box of potpourri to me once, and I carried it with me for years until I lost it somewhere in my travels.

POMANDER BALLS

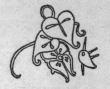

Unlike the lusty scented pomanders Queen Elizabeth wore around her neck and waist, these are more simply made with oranges and cloves.

Sister Cheryl's Pomander

Pick an orange with a fairly thick skin, or it may tear when the cloves are stuck into it. Put cloves close together all over the orange until it's completely covered. Place the cloved orange in a dish containing equal amounts of cinnamon, sandalwood, and orris root (traditionally used as a fixative for fragrances, as are benzoin, musk, and ambergris). Leave the fruit in the mixture, rolling it around every day, until it is completely dried out. Tie a ribbon around it and hang in the closet to scent your clothes. These pomanders make lovely gifts. My sister Cheryl made pomanders one Christmas and gave one each to me, my Aunt Myrtle, and my other sister, Teresa.

FRAGRANCE PILLOWS

Once, before chemical soporifics were readily available, people put tiny pillows filled with dried flowers and spices under their heads at night to induce sleep. There is sense to this. My friend Jinny planted lilac bushes under her bedroom window, claiming they not only had an aphrodisiac effect but also lulled her to sleep.

Rose Leaf Pillow

This is a very old recipe: "To well-dried rose petals and

sweet basil, add dried mint and pounded cloves. Mix well and stuff a small pillow with the mixture to induce sleep and fragrant dreams."

SACHETS

My grandmother Honor Maude used to make lemon verbena sachets, which she gave to all her grandchildren. The mixture was tied into yellow calico with scarlet ribbons.

Honor Maude's Lemon Verbena Sachet
Use pinking shears to cut circles of calico 4 inches in diameter. In the center of each circle place 1 tablespoon lemon verbena leaves, 4 to 5 orris root chips, and a piece of cotton soaked in lemon oil if you want the scent to be stronger. Tie up the lot with scarlet ribbons. Other dried flowers or leaves, such as lavender, roses, and orange blossoms, are used to make sachets too, but lemon verbena was my grandmother's favorite.

Lavender Flower Sachet
Sachets of lavender flowers with small quantities of orris root and cloves added are said to keep away moths while imparting a delicate fragrance to clothes. Mix a heaping tablespoon of lavender flowers with 4 or 5 orris root chips, and ribbon-tie the mixture in a pretty calico circle or square of cloth.

Herbal Moth Sachets
This recipe is recommended by the herbal shop Aphrodisia: Take equal parts rosemary, tansy, thyme, mint, and southernwood and a little ground cloves. Put the mixture into cloth bags and place them among clothes to ward off moths.

INCENSE

Incense is a substance that produces a pleasing aroma when burned. It is one of the oldest of fragrances. In ancient times as today it was used at religious rituals. More recently it has been used at marijuana ceremonies to mask the odor of the weed. The oldest ingredients for incense are frankincense and myrrh. Here they are used in a special recipe.

Christmas Incense

Blend together 2 ounces myrrh, 10 ounces frankincense, and 5 ounces benzoin. Burn the incense on charcoal.

MAGICAL FRAGRANCES

In the sixteenth century it was thought that certain perfumes had the power to make men speak and walk in their sleep and do wicked deeds that they would never do when awake. They were reputed to see strange unworldly sights and hear horrid sounds. These perfumes seem to have had the power of hallucinogens or the drug that turned Dr. Jekyll into Mr. Hyde, but more likely the recipes are merely good rainy day reading.

Magic Perfume No. 1

"A perfume made of Hempseeds, Fleawort seeds, Violett root too and parsley; or, a mixture of Violet root and wild Parsley makes men see into the future."

Magic Perfume No. 2

"Coriander, Henbane and the skin that is inside the Pomegranite causes men to see visions in the air and elsewhere."

THE LAST WORD ON FRAGRANCES

To scent stationery place a sheet of white paper soaked in perfume in a box of it.

To scent lingerie put your favorite essence in the rinse water.

To scent a room put a essential oil on a turned-on lightbulb or in the melted wax of a lighted candle.

To keep cool on a hot day cover yourself with an icy-cold fragrance that has been kept in the refrigerator.

To give staying power to your fragrance, soak a piece of cotton with it to put in your bra, or apply it on pulse spots, where your body is warmest: inside your wrists, in the crooks of your elbows, behind your ears, in back of your knees, at your temples, and between your breasts. Since dry skin doesn't hold fragrance as well as oily does, it's best if you have that kind of skin to wear an essential oil or a combination of them, so that the scent will cling to you.

Furthermore:
The Oriental Harems
Made
This Lip Gloss

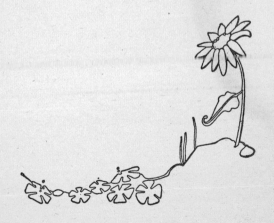

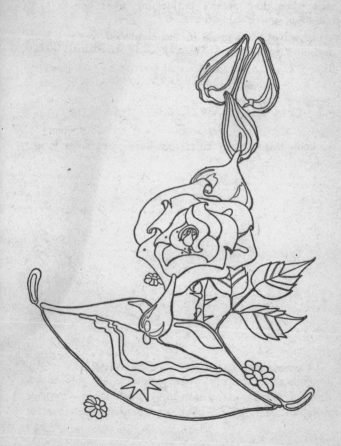

During those dark, lusty days when harems were a part of palace life (they still are in some places, I do believe), veiled women gathered to dampen a pound of heady Damask rose petals with a cup of sweet vanilla-spiked cream, forcing the lot through a piece of filmy gauze to make a substance similar to lip gloss. The pound of rose petals serviced the lips of a harem's worth of girls, but as the desirable sweet pink lip salve didn't keep well, it had to be made fresh each day, an endeavor that occupied the girls when they weren't performing scarf dances and other duties.

Lip salves were made in the eighteenth century and during Victorian times too, although well-bred ladies denied wearing them, pawning the rosy tint off as their own natural color. The contention of Victorian ladies was that their gentlemen shrank back "with disgust from the idea of kissing a pair of painted lips." Well, *somebody* then wore lip gloss, whether colored or uncolored; we know this because the recipes have come down to us.

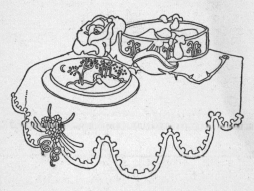

German Lip Salve (Untinted)

Melt about 1 teaspoon cocoa butter. To it add a few drops of your favorite scent. Apply this to the lips to make them soft and shiny. The least expensive container for this concoction and other lip salves is a bottle top, sealed shut with plastic wrap and a rubber band. To be fancy look for tiny lidded containers at the dime store. A nice concomitant of making your own cosmetics is finding or making pretty containers and even giving the packaged preparations as gifts.

Rose Salve (Tinted)

Mix 2 tablespoons almond oil with 1 tablespoon melted beeswax. Let this sit for 1 day. Add enough powdered alkanet root to achieve the desired shade. Tie the mixture up in muslin or cheesecloth and place it in a bowl. Leave for a day and let the alkanet slowly permeate the ointment and the whole mixture seep through the cloth into the bowl. When the mixture is cool (the beeswax was warmed to melt it), add a few drops of rose or any fragrance you prefer. Use the salve to soften and give a slight tint to the lips.

Alkanet Rouge

Add 1 part melted cocoa butter to 8 parts petroleum jelly. Mix in enough powdered alkanet to make the ointment the desired color. Tie the mixture up in muslin or cheesecloth and let it seep through into a bowl for a day. Use the rouge sparingly on cheeks to give them a blush.

Burnished Henna Cheek Color

For a natural brownish tint the women of India touch up their cheeks with a tiny bit of powdered henna.

Face Glosses

The preceding recipes are for old-fashioned methods of

adding color to the face; recently I discovered a very simple way to make lip gloss, eye gloss, and cheek gloss. A smidge of petroleum jelly or talc is spread out on a glass or pottery saucer. Drops of food coloring are added to it and stirred in with a wooden ice cream stick until the desired color is reached. I like to mix yellow and red food colorings together to get a more-orange-than-red shade for my lips and cheeks. Green-colored talc (there's blue, turquoise, chartreuse, toast, and violet too) goes on my eyes. It's a personal preference, but I like using talc rather than petroleum jelly as my base simply because it seems more controllable and less shiny on my face.

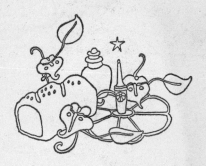

Do you know what joy it gives me to beat the cosmetics industry completely? Try it, and you'll find out.

These days we've returned to personal craftsmanship, making everything from bread and jam to patchwork quilts and clothes; why not also make hand lotions, hair rinses, and even makeup? Just as any woman who sews examines seams in storebought clothes, turns up her nose in a huff, and says, "I can do better, cheaper," you can sniff around cosmetics counters and say the same. Homemade beauty preparations are fun to make. They give you independence. They cost but a few pennies. And better yet, they work.

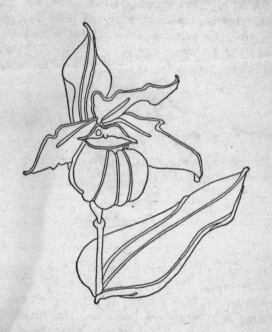

Appendix

The following firms provide free mail-order catalogs, which you can check for ingredients:

Aphrodisia Products, Inc., 28 Carmine St.,
New York, N.Y. 10014

Caswell-Massey Co., Ltd., 518 Lexington Ave.,
New York, N.Y. 10017

Herb Products Co., 11012 Magnolia Blvd.,
North Hollywood, Calif. 91601

Indiana Botanic Gardens, Inc., Hammond, Ind. 46325

Meadowbrook Herb Garden, Wyoming, R.I. 02898

Nature's Hub Co., 281 Ellis St.,
San Francisco, Calif. 94102

Index

173

179

ABOUT THE AUTHOR

DONNA LAWSON has been a beauty and fashion writer for several years for such publications as *Eye* magazine and the *New York Daily News*. She is the author of *Beauty Is No Big Deal* and *Brothers and Sisters All Over This Land*.

Facts at Your Fingertips!

How's Your Health?

Bantam publishes a line of informative books, written by top experts to help you toward a healthier and happier life.

FREE!
Bantam Book Catalog

It lists over a thousand money-saving best-sellers originally priced from $3.75 to $15.00 —bestsellers that are yours now for as little as 50¢ to $2.95!

The catalog gives you a great opportunity to build your own private library at huge savings!

So don't delay any longer—send for your catalog TODAY! It's absolutely FREE!
